Eczema

The inside view

Published in 2022 by NewGenne Limited.

Registered office of publisher:

4 Hereward Way Business Park, Harling Road, Roudham, Norfolk, NR16 2SR

United Kingdom.

This book is a 2nd edition of the original Eczema The inside view

Library of Congress Cataloging-in-Publication Data

Amblin, Bethan

Eczema The inside view

ISBN 978-0-9569707-7-0

A catalogue record of this book is available from the British Library.

Set in Bookman by Ian Taylor – www.taylorthorneprint.co.uk.

Printed in Great Britain by Taylor Thorne Print Limited, UK.

This book was produced in collaboration with Write Business Results Limited. For more information on their business book, blog and podcast services, please visit www.writebusinessresults.com or contact the team via info@writebusinessresults.com.

WRITE BUSINESS RESULTS

ECZEMA

THE INSIDE VIEW

(How you can escape eczema)

SECOND EDITION

BETHAN AMBLIN

Foreword by

Professor Terrence J Ryan DM FRCP

DEDICATION

To everyone still stuck in the eczema trap, like I once was.
There is hope.

ACKNOWLEDGEMENTS

I owe the greatest thanks to Dr Harley Farmer, for offering me the opportunity to write this book in the first place. Without him, quite literally, there would be no book, and I would not have had the tool to help so many people.

Thank you to my parents, Kath and Gareth, for supporting me along the way, and filling in the gaps of information I could not remember.

And thank you to Jacob, for being a human thesaurus and keeping me going along the journey.

CONTENTS

FOREWORD

Throughout my dermatology career I have looked at skin from the outside. Simultaneously, I have looked with keen interest at any multi-disciplinary approach which might assist with intransigent problems like atopic eczema. Yet something has been clearly missing as eczema continued to blight so many lives around the world.

For many years I have watched as Dr Harley Farmer, a veterinary surgeon by training, developed his thoughts on eczema being a matter of choice. He was bringing the field of psychology to the study of eczema and shares my desire to give Nature every chance to help us improve lives. I was aware of how he guided Bethan Amblin on from her childhood eczema. To see their association evolve into this book by a schoolgirl he helped on from eczema 10 years before is enlightening.

The true power of *Eczema The inside view* lies in how the inside view can be used so easily beside the existing outside view. The two are complimentary and in combination become greater than either one alone.

I commend this book to all with an interest in atopic eczema. It might even reveal the clue we've been missing, the clue which provides the new choice of ending eczema proactively within weeks without drugs. Let nature do it!

Professor Terence J Ryan DM FRCP

INTRODUCTION

For a schoolgirl to create a work of this depth and clarity is extraordinary. It is with immense humility and admiration that I offer the introduction to Bethan's book.

Skin is a very complicated organ and eczema brings additional complexity. I have spent almost half a century of professional life studying thousands of peer-reviewed articles in the scientific and medical literature. For all that time I've known personally what it is to live with eczema-prone skin; to always know how easily something can trigger the red itchy patches in skin we call eczema. Yet having eczema just because you have eczema-prone skin is a matter of choice. If you want to move on from eczema, you will want to do something different. Different brings hope, and this book epitomises hope.

It arose from Bethan seeking work experience in the holidays prior to beginning her final year of school. She was not commissioned to write this book. Nor was she paid to do so. However, she will earn royalties from any sales, which may ease the huge financial burden of studying medicine in England. If her book achieves the success it deserves, any financial gain from royalties will be a justified reward.

Simplicity is what this book brings to the extensive eczema literature. The numerous aspects that make up the complexity are handled with clarity through Bethan's unique writing style. The complex components are there, yet *Eczema The inside view* flows with ease.

A significant challenge for this young author was to satisfy a very diverse readership:

1. The primary intended audience is other school students. Bethan's style has to engage them, bringing as many as possible to the realisation that they have a choice of whether to keep having eczema. Graphics have been inserted into the text so people who dislike reading blocks of text can still receive the intended message by skimming the pages and only looking at the graphics.

2. Parents of those students have immense relevance, as parental support for a child progressing through the EXeczema® journey is incredibly valuable. Bethan's style needs to engage the parents in a way that allows them to provide maximum assistance.

3. Head teachers and their staff seek to reduce mental health burdens in those they teach. Eczema is one of the causes of mental health challenges which can be addressed quickly and easily throughout a school with the facts shared here. The book must resonate with the educators if they are to utilise it to best effect.

4. Medical authorities will be reading this book when the eczema public gives it the level of social status it warrants. To earn medical support this book must be scientifically and medically credible, which is why Bethan has cited references in the text. The bibliography in the appendix provides confidence for the authorities that they will find credibility garnered from their own evidence-based literature.

Some have said Bethan is a lucky girl to have been given the opportunity to write this book. Was it luck that brought Bethan to be in the right place at the right time? I believe luck arises when opportunity meets preparedness. Eczema is very common around the world, so the opportunity was always there. Preparedness is another matter entirely. I recall how Bethan's eyes lit up when I asked if she wanted to write this book. I used my psychology skills to delve deep in search of any reservations in her young psyche. What I found was her high level of preparedness. Luck, through opportunity meeting determined preparedness, was then supplemented with her eagerness to help others.

I hope *Eczema The inside view* brings Bethan all the luck she deserves. I suspect she will judge the level of success by how many people of all ages come to their own realisations of where the cure for their eczema lies. Be ready to look beyond the patches of red itchy skin. This is, after all, the *inside view*.

Dr Harley Farmer PhD BVSc(Hons) BVBiol(Path) MRCVS

CHAPTER 1

MY STORY

Why would I go to the trouble of writing this book? To share something few people with eczema know, and to help people explain eczema to themselves, their families, friends and perhaps their doctors.

I plan for several different groups of people to read this book and benefit from it, the first being the group that I once fell in: eczema sufferers. You've tried all the creams out there – those prescribed, found in drugstores, even the ones you've heard about on the internet. Nothing's working and you're desperate; eczema is beginning to take over your life. You could have been told from a young age that this is something that cannot be cured, you just have to wait to grow out of it, that there's nothing that can be done. This may not sit right with you. Surely there must be something that can be done?

Another group is the parents of these desperate children. Like them, you are desperate yourself. Eczema runs in your genetics; you may even be feeling guilty about your struggling child. Doctors and hospital trips have become second nature. Surely there must be another way?

Then there are the teachers at schools. You have seen the devastation and distraction as a consequence of eczema in young children. The distinctive disease puts them at a disadvantage to other healthy children with "normal" skin. You've noticed that they're distracted from schoolwork and aren't as cheerful as the others. But, if you're not from a medical background, there's nothing you can do, right?

The final group of people I hope to help with this book are the doctors and GPs who are all too familiar with eczema. Countless young people have come in to see you and been sent away with creams, only to then come back asking for more help. You may have noticed that in the years to come, these are the same people who come back for reasons relating to their mental health. But that's just a coincidence – there couldn't have been anything that you could have done, right?

All of those perspectives are right if you wish to retain the *outside view* of eczema. When you appreciate the *inside view*, I suggest you will find a new source of confidence. You may even choose to do something different. I have written this book to share the information I wish I had always known, to ensure that the countless other children suffering have the opportunity to make an informed decision about their skin, their lives.

Throughout the book, you will see quotations from the text as bold inserts, because some of the intended readers may show little interest in reading blocks of text. The inserts allow them to skim the book and still gain the essential knowledge. They would gain more if they were to read the text in full, but first I must help them to take sufficient interest.

We'll start with the good news: I can say I am free from eczema, free from the creaming regimes, free from hospital trips. At the age of eight, I was liberated. That is to say, I am not completely eczema free. Occasionally it will come back, predominantly in the creases of my elbows and knees, but I know my triggers and how to resolve it. I avoid the word cured in relation to skin as it's so controversial, but you could say I have been cured from the mindset of "this will never go away".

"... cured from the mindset..."

My first sign of eczema was rolling my ankles and wrists in circles as a baby. Being my parents' first child, they understandably thought it was simply a sweet thing babies did. Little did they know it was a consequence of the eczema; I was trying to scratch. At only 18 months, my parents were buying moisturisers from chemists in an attempt to control the patches of dry skin, which were ever present throughout my time as a toddler. Then, as I joined primary school aged four, the redness and itchiness started to become more intense; and so began the doctors and hospital trips, and the emollients (medicinal moisturisers) and steroid creams, entering me into the perpetual cycle of worsening eczema and stronger creams, lasting many years.

"Have you been swimming?" was the question I was asked as a child, more times than I'd like to admit, due to my wet look caused by the prescribed emollients having been slathered upon me numerous times a day. I'd go to bed in "magic pyjamas" – wet bandages covering me head to toe, with a dry layer over the top, to help my skin retain water. My life was a tick-box of treatments, and it felt as if almost as soon as the first box was ticked, the next started. It took sticker-charts and rewards to persuade me to comply. It was life consuming – not just for me, but also my parents. On top of requiring over an hour daily to tend to my needs, when it came to planning trips away, it became such a logistical challenge to either bring all my treatments with us or create detailed plans for carers, that trips became rarities. For one weekend trip away, we would need the pyjamas, the emollients, the steroid creams, the reward charts, the antihistamine, the oats for the bath, the ice packs, the mittens to stop me scratching… it would all have to come.

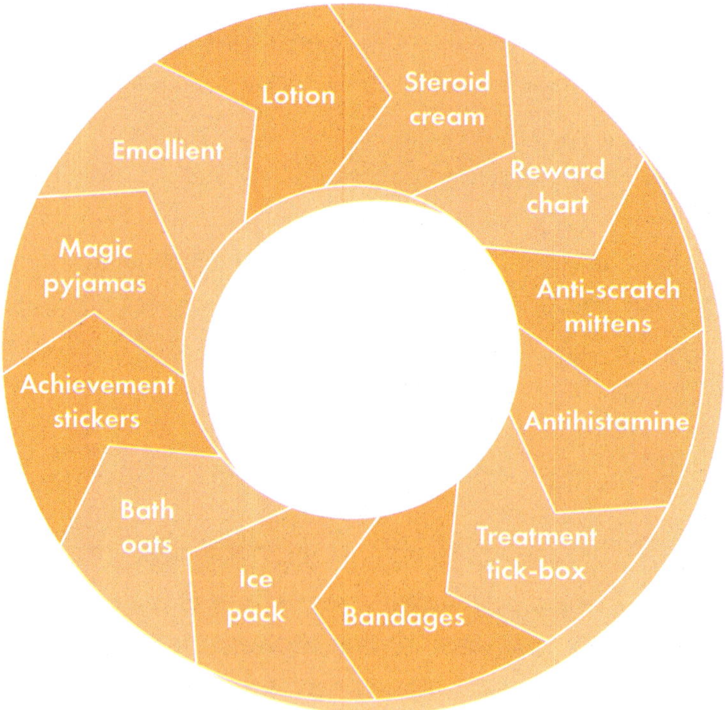

To help support all of us, we joined the local hospital's eczema support group, to gain ideas on treatments and share experiences. But most importantly, the group reminded us that we weren't the only ones; that there were always people around us who understood and could empathise with what we were going through. It was there we first met Dr Harley (his full name is actually Dr Harley Farmer, but as a small child I always called him Dr Harley, and he's happy that I continue to do so in this book). He was giving a presentation on his new ideas about the relation of prescribed eczema treatments and the maintenance of eczema.[1][2] Dry, eczema-prone skin contains cracks which allow foreign material to penetrate the skin barrier. The immune system uses inflammation to expel the foreign substances. In summary, he told us the creams prescribed were a factor in the inflammation and itchiness of my skin. He was describing toxicology.

TOXICOLOGY

Toxicology is the study of the adverse effects of chemical substances on living organisms.

With my mother being a medical professional herself, she could understand the science behind Dr Harley's reasoning. She used her own knowledge to debate whether stopping the use of my prescribed treatments was something we could do with success. That, and the desperation we all felt while trapped in this cycle of treatment and inflammation, pushed the decision of following Dr Harley to help with my eczema.

It was a tough and, quite frankly, scary decision: whether to follow the official medical advice with my treatment routine, despite it being clearly damaging; or, now that we were aware of the facts, to stop following medical advice and completely stop using their products. Yet, when my mother looked back, it seemed obvious that if the prescribed treatments weren't damaging, then they would have helped my eczema. The multiple years that I had been religiously using them with no avail proved that something different had to be done, and that something different was to test Dr Harley's ideas.

In showing interest, he educated us on why my eczema was persisting. It was a combination of multiple factors: from the creams I used damaging my skin, to the creams disrupting my natural skin cycle of flushing out unwanted substances, and creating unnatural environments for different bacteria to grow, even to the belief I had held, having had eczema my whole life, that it couldn't be cured. Dr Harley showed us a way out.

Using Dr Harley's gentle foam wash and oil-free emollient, allowed my skin to break the eczema cycle and heal itself.

"There were no prescription drugs."

There were no prescription drugs. There were no reactive chemicals that damaged new skin cells. There were no heavy lotions giving me a greasy look. My body had the opportunity to heal itself, and my mind had the chance to bring my confidence back. I am still the same person, with the same skin, same genes. I can go places and do things now that would have once triggered inflammation in my eczema. My success arose from the realisation that my eczema was a trap and that I could escape the trap, breaking the cycle and following a path to normal skin.

"I have escaped the misery of eczema.

I've spent a decade examining how I achieved something so amazing.

If you have eczema, or care for someone with it, please be ready for the amazing.

Through this book, I seek to help others and I seek your help to achieve it all."

I can look back at the child I was, smothered in different creams and emollients every morning and every night, and think, "I wish I had known what I know now." And for everyone who doesn't know, here is my chance to help to educate you about the choices you have regarding your skin, just like Dr Harley did for us.

When I had eczema, my skin was protecting me; now I protect my skin.

That single sentence warrants a paragraph of its own. It sounds simple and logical yet it encompasses so much. It emphasises how the red inflammatory process I called eczema was the correct and desired protective response against something being put on the outside of my skin. Through its use of inflammation, my skin was protecting me from outside products. If the chemicals in those products had been benign, there would have been no reason for my skin to react and protect me. Applying the products was deemed to be normal. I know now the way the skin reacted was equally normal.

Yet, at the time, I felt my skin was reacting against me. I believed the red inflammation on the outside was ruling my life. Ironically it was the placing of those products on my skin that ruled my life, and the redness was a clue. For years we lacked the perspective to use that simple clue. We chose to fear the clue rather than use it to my advantage. Changing that perspective, that view, was like flicking a light switch. Which is why I can now protect my skin.

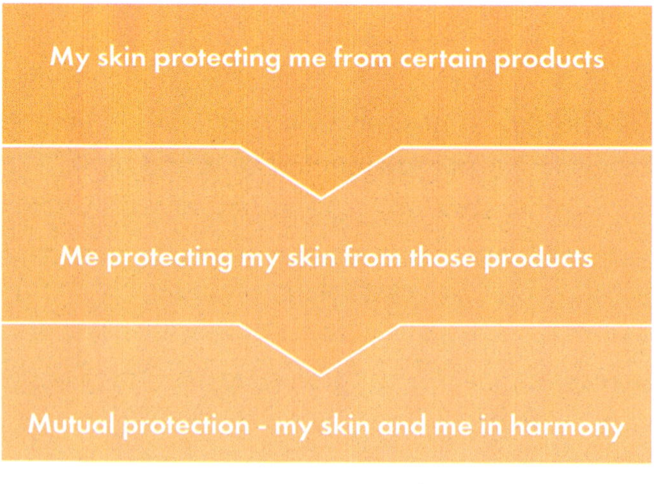
My skin protecting me from certain products
Me protecting my skin from those products
Mutual protection - my skin and me in harmony

As time goes on, and technology improves, industries have the capability to include many chemicals which theoretically help the skin. Yet, all the skin wants is to be natural. It has evolved, by itself, to do its job of keeping your inside in and the outside out. I protect it by using very gentle skincare products. It protects me by doing its job.

Writing this book allows me to help people with eczema around me. I don't like to discuss my escape with them in case they choose to feel even more helpless. Yet from years of living with, and combatting eczema, I know that the key to having wonderful skin – the skin Nature intended us to have – is being able to explain eczema. And who better to guide people to their own realisations than someone who has experienced all of this? I spent so much of my early life just accepting that I would live with the misery of eczema, until someone offered to share this knowledge.

Eczema is complicated; throughout the book there will be bubbles of explanations of different "ologies" and their relation to eczema. You will meet seven of them, and you will have seen the toxicology bubble already. Some may notice that dermatology, the study of the skin, is absent from the list. Eczema is defined as a skin condition; it is shown in the skin, yet it is actually the skin trying to defend the person. Knowing that becomes the key.

The last chapter of the book provides an indication of the fun we have in being part of the community that has arisen around Dr Harley's sharing nature. One of the things I admire about him is how he openly admits he is still learning about eczema and the ways people react to it – and so am I. He likes to suggest that we keep learning and read with an open mind, as every person has something to teach and something to share.

Finally, the bibliography at the end lists the sources and references used to support what I present in this book. A bracketed number in the text, like [17], refers to reference number 17 in the bibliography. It is an indication of what material I have used to justify my statement. I say this in the first chapter so you can read in confidence knowing which of my comments have full medical credibility. When the source is a website, it must be accepted that the content of the site may change. The points I quote from websites are those available in early 2022. If there is no bracketed number after a comment, that comment is the best I have been able to find amongst the generally held beliefs. The equivalent valid medical reference may exist; I just haven't found it yet among the multitude of references available.

Using and trusting my points and references will allow you to understand eczema, and once that has been done, you will earn a new choice: the choice of doing something different. With me as a prime example, you will already know that doing more of the same will achieve more of the same. If you dare to hope for wonderful skin, you can dare to do something different.

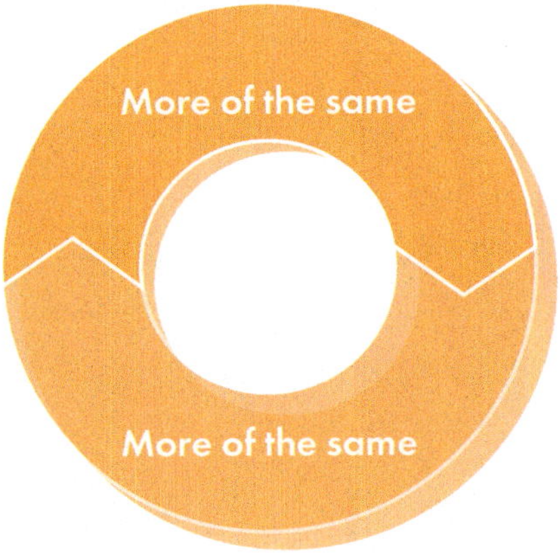

OR

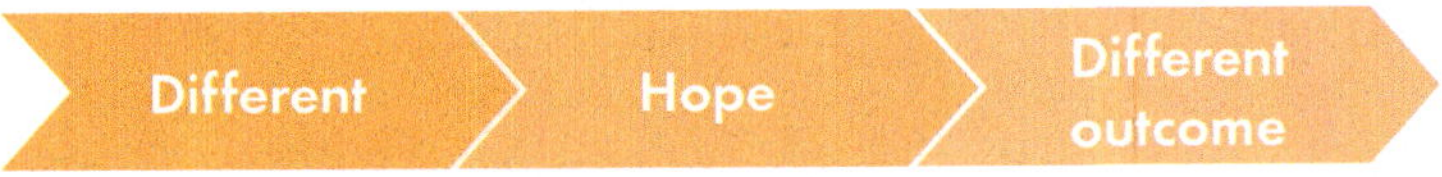

Reading this book and sharing with others are great ways to begin.

CHAPTER 2

INTRODUCTION TO ATOPIC ECZEMA

I'll begin with the facts and figures to help you to understand eczema more clearly. It is generally accepted that 10% of adults in the UK have eczema, with 20% of babies being diagnosed with eczema within their first year, with me being one of them. It is also widely accepted that eczema is a "condition of the affluent". In poorer countries it is rarer, while being common in wealthy nations like the UK. This could be explained by the better medical services here being able to detect and diagnose it – or could equally be explained by the treatments so frequently prescribed, causing irritation.

Similarly, it has also been accepted that in the 1950s atopic eczema was rare, and diagnoses have been increasing ever since. Again it could be due to the same reasons as above. Eczema could be called a disease of our time and culture, a bit like obesity. A good example of a treatment leading to disease would be the widespread use of opiate antidepressants last century. Many people were prescribed the treatments, and only time allowed the medical profession to appreciate that the resultant addictions eventually became a bigger problem than the depression they were intended to cure. The products were prescribed with good intent and a subsequent change in perspective showed the real effect.

The actual definition of eczema is one that frequently changes. After being a common condition for more than 50 years, you would hope there would be more clarity. Yet as we learn more about eczema, it seems definitions vary depending on where you look. I for one know that having so many definitions can leave you so confused you actually end up with none to use. When friends asked what was wrong with me, often I could not even reply. Some say, "that when AE [atopic eczema] is very active, it may become moist and weep and small water blisters may develop."[3] Many others fail to mention the blisters. Many definitions refer to genetic anomalies, with one specifically saying, "In atopic eczema, dry skin is due to a genetically defective skin barrier."[4] One source goes beyond the cause and mentions that when eczema is active, "irritating substances enter the skin, causing itching and inflammation."[5] The same authors say, "Approximately one third of children with AE will also develop asthma and/or hay fever." A dictionary definition includes, "areas of skin become red, rough and sore and make you want to scratch them."[6]

Bearing in mind that when most people refer to eczema, they mean atopic eczema, you might understand the conflict in the definitions. Conflict only seeds confusion over the matter. Confusion leads to using differing methods to manage eczema: methods that won't all work and subsequently lead to a belief that you cannot positively end eczema.

The primary aim of writing this book is to help readers better understand their eczema. This in turn gives them the opportunity to take the information on board and make informed choices to help themselves. So Dr Harley and I would like to offer a simpler definition: eczema is the state of confusion over red skin.

"... state of confusion over red skin."

Confusion is just as big a component of eczema as the red skin. So we seek to bring confusion to the fore as a means of enabling a change in mindset. A change in mindset arising from a changed perspective is often easier to instil than a change in the repeated action of applying the same products every day. I know from my own experience how the routine of applying all those products had become a habit. It was a change in mindset that allowed us to look back on the confusion as a means of moving on from eczema. So this deliberately simplistic definition of eczema helps people appreciate there is something they can do easily and quickly. In effect, eczema becomes a choice; you can choose to have eczema or you can choose to move on from it.

"... you can choose to have eczema or you can choose to move on from it."

Eczema also has genetic factors. Having two parents with atopic eczema increases the susceptibility for the child to develop eczema by 90%.[7] That said, this is a factor, not a cause. It increases the chances of developing eczema when an irritant is applied to the skin. In contrast, if the products being applied are not irritants, then there is no opportunity for eczema to develop. These choices will be made very clear as this book progresses. This is something I have learnt myself. Having naturally eczema-prone skin, I could have the mindset of acceptance, as I have a tendency for eczema in my genes so I will always have eczema. However, the reality is that without any cause for irritation, my tendency towards eczema has become null. My eczema has gone.

It might help at this stage to discuss sunburn. In contrast to people with black skin, those with white skin have a genetic makeup which makes them prone to sunburn. However, having sunburn-prone skin does not mean they need to have sunburn. Only when they take actions that allow sunburn to occur, does their skin turn red. Genes make a person prone to sunburn; but their actions result in sunburn. Genes make a person prone to eczema; but their actions result in eczema.

"Genes make a person prone to sunburn; but their actions result in sunburn.

Genes make a person prone to eczema; but their actions result in eczema."

Another significant genetic factor in eczema is the number of filaggrin gene copies.[8] Most people with normal skin have 12 copies of the gene, and their skin cells make the correct number of granules which allow them to make a strong skin barrier. These granules are vital in the understanding of eczema, which makes this a good time to show why we know they exist. It arose with the introduction of histology.

HISTOLOGY

Histology, also known as microscopic anatomy or microanatomy, is the branch of biology that studies the microscopic anatomy of biological tissues.

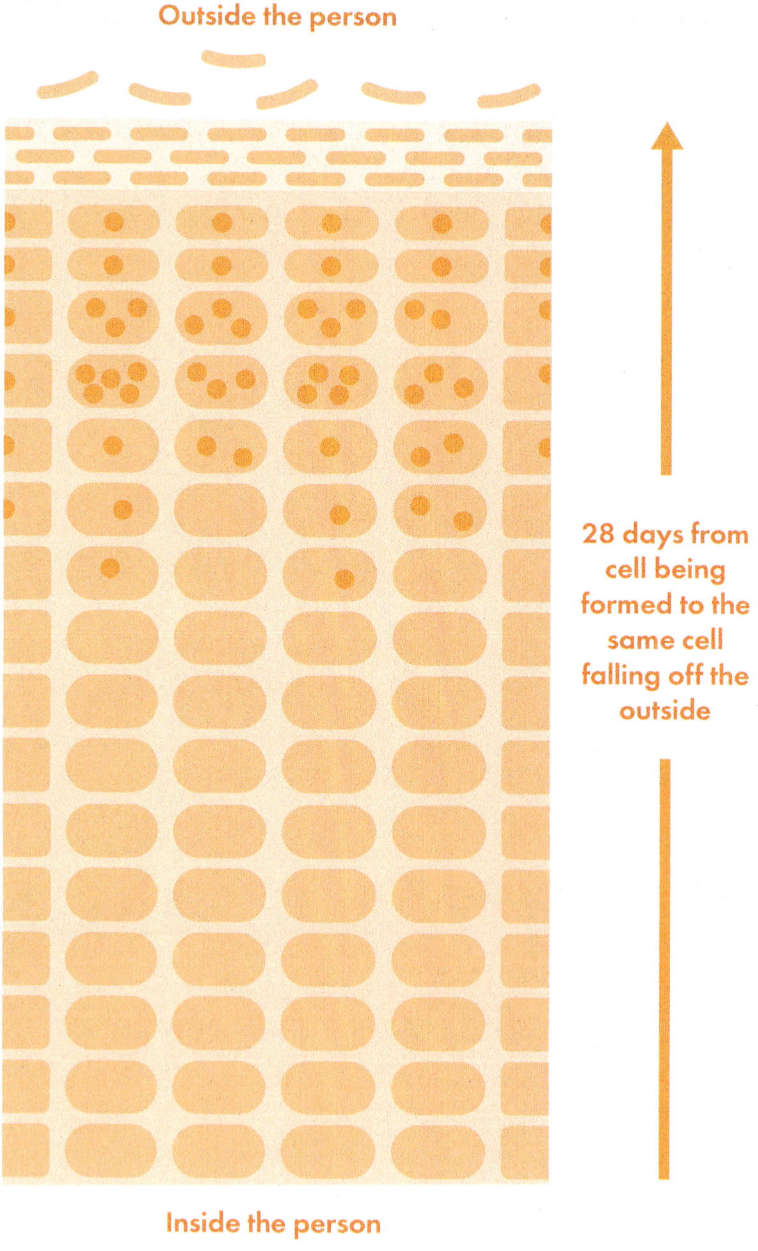
Outside the person
28 days from cell being formed to the same cell falling off the outside
Inside the person

You will see this schematic diagram of the epidermal cells repeatedly as I emphasise different aspects. The dots shown in some cells represent the granules which include the material made when the filaggrin gene was read. Filaggrin is a protein which aligns fibres in epidermal cells.

People with 11 copies make fewer of the granules in their skin cells, and those with just 10 copies make even fewer. It is rare, but there are a few people who have no copies of the filaggrin gene. This causes *ichthyosis vulgaris,* a condition which causes skin to appear like fish scales.[9] Without a strong skin barrier, many modern-day products containing foreign chemicals can penetrate the skin barrier and induce an inflammatory response.[10]

Despite it being fairly rare to have fewer than 12 filaggrin gene copies, many children are tested for these defects in an attempt to explain inflammation contributing towards their eczema.[11] This sometimes leads to acceptance that they will forever have eczema. Still, you cannot become inflamed without a cause for that. All too often, this cause will be external products. Even with genetic factors, with natural conditions your skin can heal.

How is eczema treated?

Multiple therapies are used to treat and manage eczema. There are the first prescribed moisturisers, emollients, ointments, steroid creams, lotions, skin washes, antihistamines… the list could continue forever. Then, for further help, herbal remedies like lavender to soothe

the skin, oat baths, dietary changes, and aloe vera are used for a more natural approach. Sometimes in severe cases wet wrapping – a layer of wet bandages underneath a layer of dry bandages – is used to keep moisture in overnight. All of these mentioned I have used at some point during my childhood with eczema, before Dr Harley offered the suggestion of looking at eczema from the inside rather than applying products on the outside.

I mention how many skin treatments can penetrate the skin through cracks and damage new skin cells; however, I must emphasise how this is only for the 10% of the population with eczema. Usually, for many with a complete skin barrier and without eczema, they work well to help the skin retain moisture. This is usually by mineral oil forming a water repellant barrier over the skin to keep the moisture in. Despite this being a widespread belief, in the 1992 mineral oil article, it was revealed that the mineral oil applied to skin actually penetrates (even healthy skin) to the depth of a few skin cells deep and locates itself between the ceramide lipid bilayers.[12]

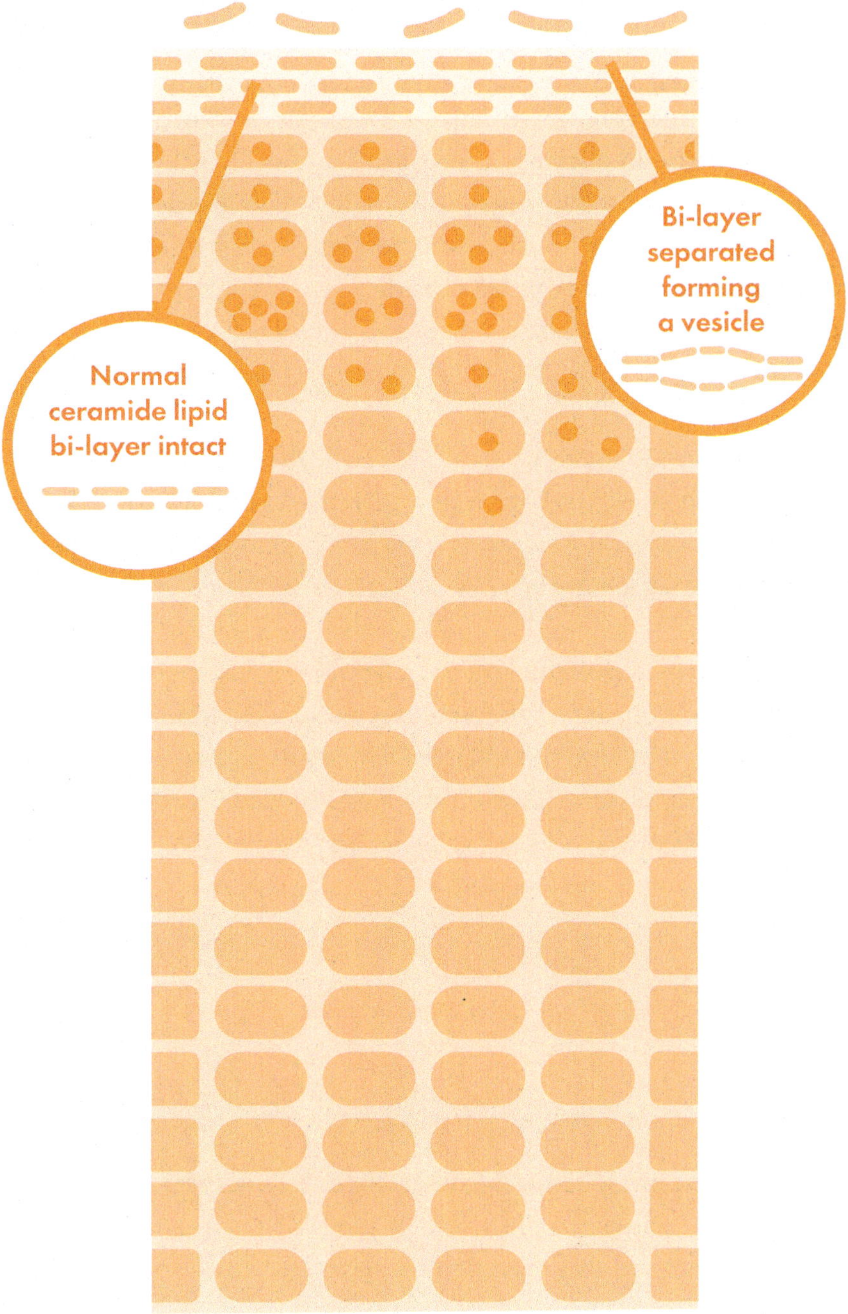
Bi-layer separated forming a vesicle
Normal ceramide lipid bi-layer intact

Many modern creams are free of mineral oil. Yet interestingly, even with the 1992 knowledge, medicinal creams with a UK Product Licence often do contain mineral oil. This will be discussed further in a subsequent chapter.

On many websites with information about eczema, it commonly says that eczema cannot be cured.[13] I spent most of my childhood believing this. And so, I applied my creams and managed my eczema. Yet, within two weeks of deciding to act upon our change in mindset, there were no noticeable patches of eczema left on my skin. Dr Harley led my mother and I to believe that there was hope it would be healed. With that hope we decided to escape our routine that maintained my eczema. And with that escape, my skin had an opportunity to heal itself.

Dr Harley makes a point of stressing he did not cure my eczema and nor did my mother. Between them they decided on a course of action which allowed my skin to heal itself. Once the skin was normal with a fully functional skin barrier, there was no need for inflammation, which is another way of saying there was no eczema. No cure was discussed, no cure was needed and no cure was used.

"... a course of action which allowed my skin to heal itself."

Having heard from so many trusted sources that eczema isn't curable, some may be accepting of the belief they will always have eczema. This can be referred to as "learned helplessness". You've got to believe it can be healed before it will heal. I was one of those people, and it did. I agree there is no one thing that can be applied to cure eczema. But with myself and the many others whose mindset Dr Harley has helped to change, allowing our skin to heal, the one common factor was the hope we had that it could be healed.

Seek a cure and eczema goes on.

Hope with no cure and eczema goes.

I know it can be hard to believe that changing one thing can heal you. I found it almost too good to be true. But I trusted what I heard we could do, and knew that the methods we were using were directed at our thinking rather than the skin. So we dived in.

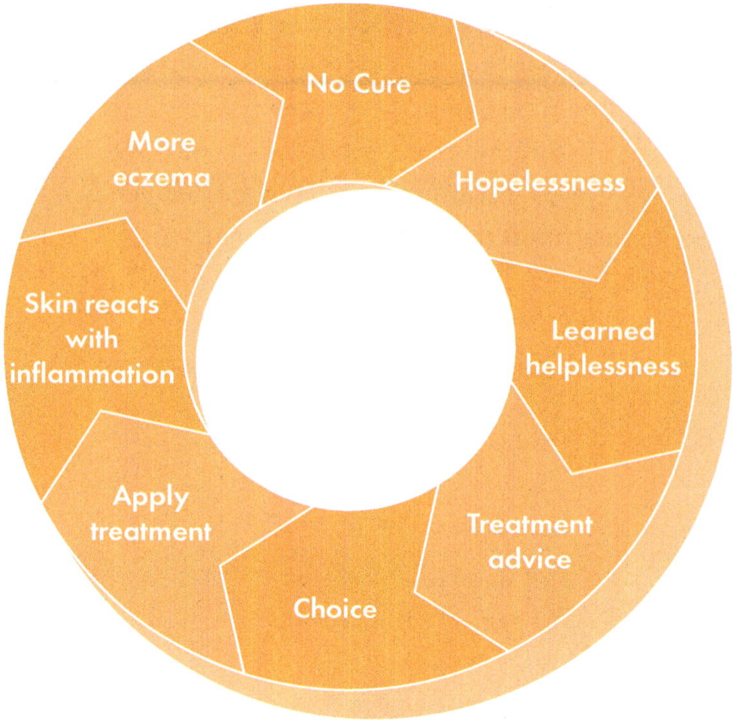

Break the cycle by doing something different at Choice

Hope is available to everyone, yet many find themselves in a state of mind that makes it very difficult to hope. When someone is in such a state of mind, it is both polite and wise to be very gentle with any suggestion of hope. It can be a step too far. More is gained by letting them reach their own realisation that hope comes from "different". They already know that if they continue doing what they have been doing, they will achieve what they have always been achieving. If they are content with such achievements, they are more likely to maintain their actions.

They may dream of having wonderful skin free from eczema, yet as we all know, dreams end when you wake up. Good dreams have a value, yet little changes when all you rely on is dreams. Something different needs to happen in order to achieve something different. Learning that hope arises from different can be a gentle introduction to the value in trying something different. The easiest first step is often a different mindset. And even easier is to learn of what happened when someone else changed their mindset. That is why personal stories like mine have such value. They do not tell people what they must do; they simply show people what could happen for them if they ventured towards trying the same mindset. By definition it will be a different mindset. That realisation introduces the word different, and if they learn the word hope is often anchored to the word different, they have begun the process. People choose how they want to react to words. If they choose to be hurt by a word, they will be hurt. In contrast if they choose to see hope in a word, the outcome will be different. Someone in a stuck state of choosing to be hurt must be allowed time to wonder if that state is serving them well. Perhaps they have a secondary gain in seeing eczema continue, in which case it is polite to leave them in that state.

"... the word hope is often anchored to the word different..."

In time, they may wish to achieve the different outcome of having eczema-free skin and that is when they may choose to read or reread this book. It is up to them. Eczema is a choice, and that choice arises from knowing there is a choice.

"Eczema is a choice, and that choice arises from knowing there is a choice."

CHAPTER 3

ATOPIC MARCH

In the article "Is atopic eczema iatrogenic?" Dr Harley asks whether the word atopic would be better replaced with iatrogenic, meaning caused by medical treatment.[1] The term atopic usually relates to antibodies. Atopic eczema sufferers will often have asthma (atopic bronchitis) or hay fever (atopic rhinitis), or both. The latter conditions are based on true antibody reactions, so the use of the word atopic is fully justified. However, Dr Harley argues that eczema is actually an irritant reaction, in which case no antibodies are involved. That is why he questioned the use of the word atopic in the name. However, if the inflammation called eczema truly is a reaction to the medicaments being applied, then a more useful medical adjective would be iatrogenic. The article questions whether medical personnel could be responsible for the maintenance of eczema.

Even though the article was published in a peer-reviewed medical journal, it gained little traction. Perhaps it was a little too controversial and uncomfortable in the medical setting. Therefore I will expand on it here as I am one of the unfortunate ones who has experienced all three of the "atopic" conditions.

"Atopic march", also known as "allergic march", is a medical term referring to onset of allergies, usually starting with eczema, with hay fever and asthma to come.

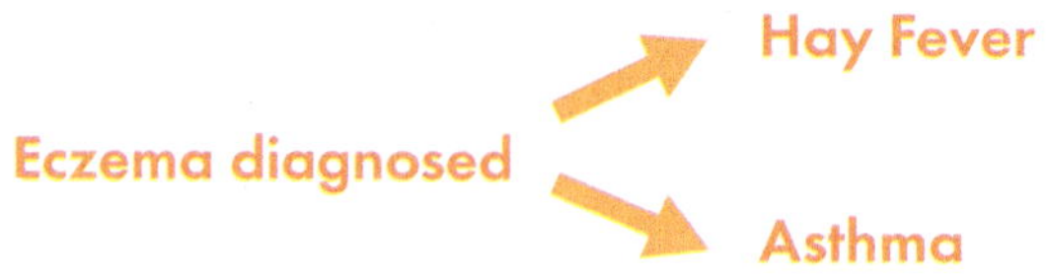

In the 20% of babies who are diagnosed with eczema, often doctors will warn the parents of this. Being told there is worse to come is understandably concerning. With the chances of developing atopic eczema being up to 90% when both the parents also have atopic conditions, feelings of empathy and even possibly guilt could be felt.

When my mother was told I had eczema as a baby, naturally she was also forewarned about the horrors to come. The only good news was that she was told that I would "grow out of it" and that there was nothing we could do apart from wait and manage it. A medical professional herself, it was dispiriting to hear that it was out of her control. She disliked the fact that all my creams – which would take hours each day in total to complete the routine – seemed as if they didn't make a difference. This repeated for years. This is why, with her knowledge, she sensed hope in Dr Harley's way of explaining eczema.

In further chapters, I will be discussing the relevance of Th2 effector cells in comparison to Th2 suppressor cells. For now, the importance of this is that when the allergens penetrate the eczema-affected skin, Th2 lymphocytes are created as an immune response. They are sent to locations where they will likely encounter the allergen again, especially the nose and lungs, as well as the gut. Then, when the allergen is encountered in the nose, hay fever symptoms will occur. Likewise, if the allergen is breathed into the lungs, asthma symptoms will occur.

IMMUNOLOGY

Immunology is the study of the immune system, and in relation to eczema, it relates to the irritant reaction to foreign chemicals that enter the skin.

The onset of hay fever and asthma after being diagnosed with eczema is often due to the damaged skin as a consequence of eczema. Healthy skin is a barrier. It keeps everything external out and everything internal in. But when inflamed skin is scratched, it breaks the barrier. Perhaps you've felt your skin weep in extreme cases – that's the barrier broken and the internal getting out. Most importantly though, in these cases it means the outside can get in. The antigens penetrate the skin barrier through the weeping areas. They travel to the lymph nodes where specialised T memory cells form. Some of these then travel to the nose and antibodies are used to combat the antigen. This is hay fever.

The important point of distinction is that eczema is an irritant response, whereas hay fever and asthma are antibody responses.

The following diagram has been adapted with Dr Harley's permission from his book *What is eczema? A path to ending the misery.*[2]

Unfortunately, as I too have experienced, even once the skin clears of eczema, the hay fever and asthma will remain. This is due to hay fever and asthma being antibody responses. Eczema is an irritant response. That distinction is vital to understanding eczema. It demonstrates why it has been asked whether atopic eczema is actually not atopic in the sense of being antibody related. Yes, if there wasn't an opportunity for the skin to become inflamed in the first place, the allergens could not have had a chance to penetrate the skin and lead to the atopic march. Allergens cannot penetrate healthy skin. Some call the broken skin of eczema "leaky skin", similar to the term "leaky gut" used with intestinal disorders. This fits when you recall the Th2 lymphocytes also localise in the gut.

This really emphasises the importance of preventing eczema, as opposed to managing it. Allergies are increasing: in the last twenty years in the UK, incidences of common allergies have trebled.[14] And with people where the root of these allergies begins with allergens getting in via eczematous skin, it makes sense to prevent eczema developing. By decreasing the huge 20% of babies who are diagnosed with eczema, it will prevent countless cases of asthma, hay fever and other allergies developing.

For now, doctors diagnosing eczema in young babies will continue to forewarn parents that there is worse to come. It is fair and proper to do so. Nothing has been changed yet to prevent it. Yet so much could be done to do so with a constructive change in mindset.

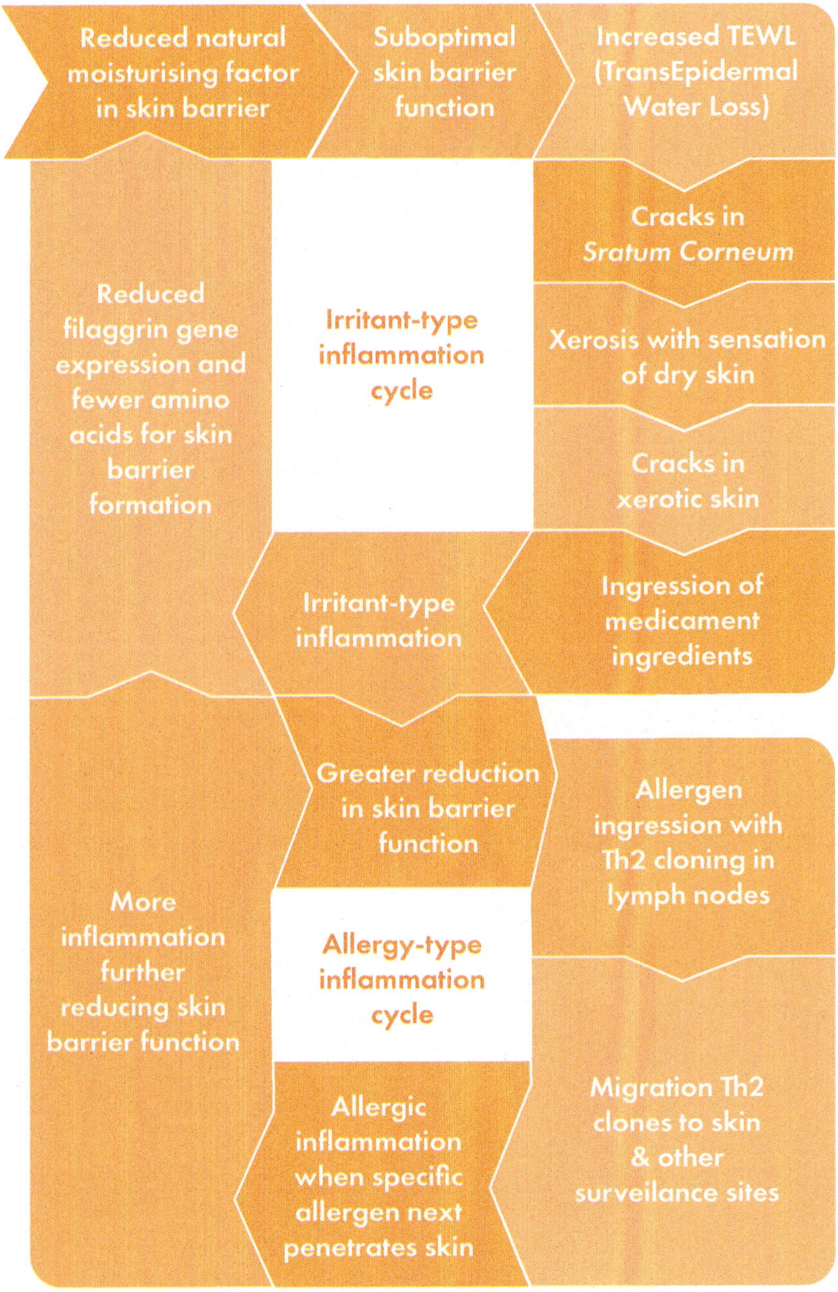
Reduced natural moisturising factor in skin barrier
Suboptimal skin barrier function
Increased TEWL (TransEpidermal Water Loss)
Cracks in *Sratum Corneum*
Xerosis with sensation of dry skin
Cracks in xerotic skin
Ingression of medicament ingredients
Irritant-type inflammation
Irritant-type inflammation cycle
Reduced filaggrin gene expression and fewer amino acids for skin barrier formation
Greater reduction in skin barrier function
Allergen ingression with Th2 cloning in lymph nodes
Migration Th2 clones to skin & other surveilance sites
Allergic inflammation when specific allergen next penetrates skin
Allergy-type inflammation cycle
More inflammation further reducing skin barrier function

CHAPTER 4

KNOWLEDGE IS KEY

There is a huge amount of information published in medical journals regarding eczema. This is done in order to share information and new finds within the medical profession.

Similarly, there are huge amounts of information available to the public on social media platforms. In my case, I was part of an eczema-support Facebook group where we would share what worked for us and other pieces of advice. These platforms were very good for advice and guidance, but pieces of medical or scientific evidence were rarely seen. And if they were seen, the short attention span so often used on social media meant they were rarely fully read and understood, for they were so long. Unfortunately this is the case with many eczema-related platforms on social media. Most contain so much word-of-mouth advice with no medical basis, that you need to sift through to find something useful. Then, if the medical publications are posted, as they are so long in comparison to the short posts of guidance, they aren't acknowledged as much as they potentially could be.

Even with so much information around you, it is hard to know what to follow.

Another downside about social platforms is that they can, and often do, turn into echo chambers. With so many like-minded people sharing information, most of it is from one perspective. Often, this perspective is of desperation and lack of understanding. Echo chambers are environments where people only encounter viewpoints similar to their own, reinforcing their own beliefs. A prime example could be an anti-vaxxer joining an anti-vaxxer group, and only choosing to hear similar opinions.

In the case of eczema, this would mean the social platform reinforcing beliefs of managing eczema, in the belief it will be present chronically. This I would refer to as "learned helplessness": the belief it will never heal, and therefore no action exists that would help it heal. Offering a suggestion that eczema can be actively ended by a change in mindset earns very negative reactions in some internet social fora. It would be a view they had not already been sharing, so it would be inappropriate to suggest it in an echo chamber where it was not welcome.

Something very similar goes for medical publications in journals. If an idea has not been published in a peer-reviewed medical journal, it is deemed to have zero credibility. Yet we all know that the absence of evidence is not the same as evidence of absence. The journals can only reveal when evidence is available. And it sometimes takes a very long time before something which is blatantly obvious to the general public warrants the cost of the research required to prove and publish it.

There's so much information on the internet, in books, journals, from the doctors. To best simplify it I will say this: the skin acts as required. If a foreign irritant is applied, the skin will react to, and work to remove, this. It keeps what's in, in and what's out, out. If it is damaged, it will try to heal. Medicine gives us the chance to aid the body to do what is natural. This has been progressed over time to allow medicines to become relied upon, as they do such a good job at the narrow, specific task they are intended to address. Yet sometimes the best thing is to step back and let the body do what it does naturally – protect you and heal itself.

A remarkable but often forgotten example is grazing a knee. The force of friction between the floor and the skin on the knee, breaks the skin barrier and the layers and layers of skin cells. The skin has rapid trauma – but is expected to heal itself, and rightly so.

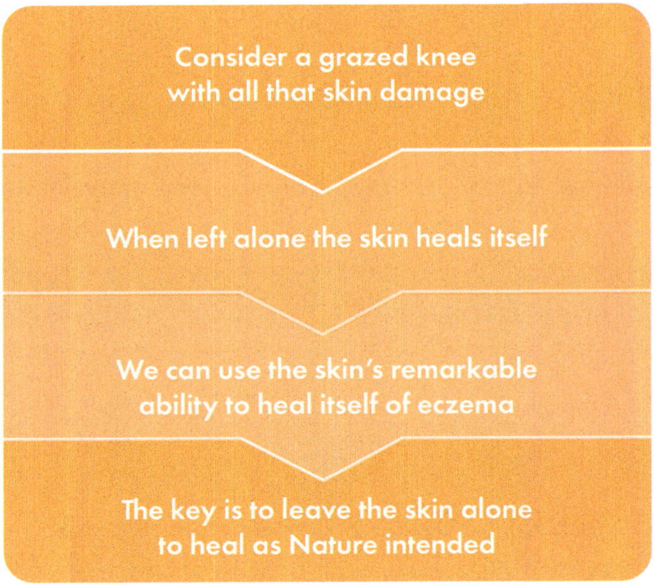
Consider a grazed knee with all that skin damage
When left alone the skin heals itself
We can use the skin's remarkable ability to heal itself of eczema
The key is to leave the skin alone to heal as Nature intended

Very rarely does eczema get so severe that a large area of the epidermis has been removed, even with severe scratching. Eczematous skin has complete potential to heal by itself. The most common reason why it doesn't is that it continues getting damaged by more irritants being applied and when scratched. Without irritation, whether that be from clothes, heat, stress, or foreign chemicals, and so no itch and inflammation, the skin will heal.

If all you hope to do is manage eczema, you already know how to do that. The medical and social platforms have taught you how to do it and you are likely to be very good at it. For some readers, you will have been doing it for decades. Sadly for some, it has been happening for generations in the same family.

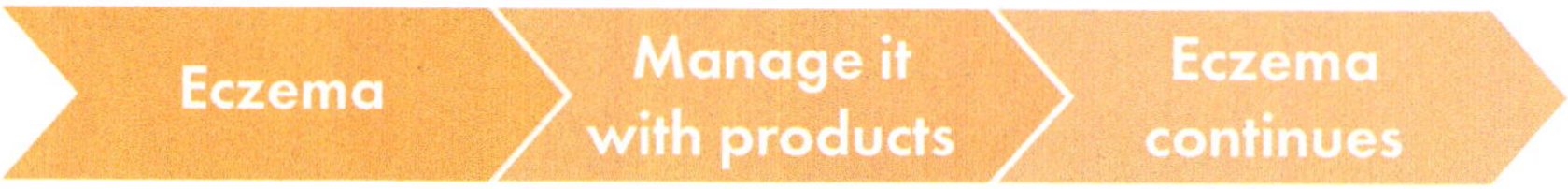

As an exercise, think back on all the advice you have relied upon to manage eczema. Now, purely in your mind, go back through the advice and replace the word *manage* with *maintain*. Do you notice how the story remains the same? In reality the two words are interchangeable. When you try to manage your eczema, you will maintain your eczema.

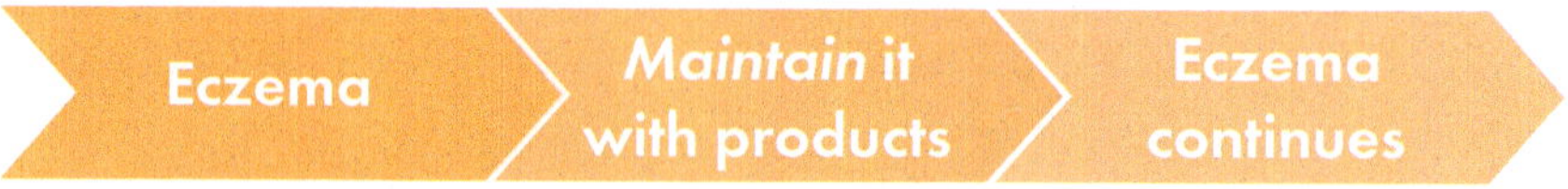

I hope this book will reveal a new choice. The title of this chapter is "Knowledge Is Key". You might ask the key to what? It is the key to something different. Psychologists often say different brings hope. Without doing something different, you deny yourself hope of achieving something different.

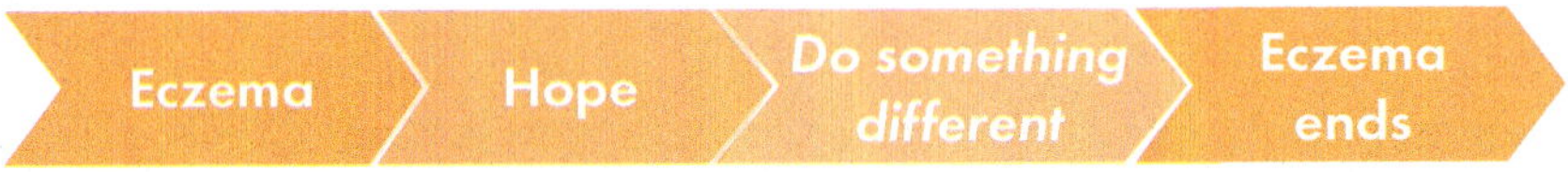

Ask yourself if you have come to your own realisation that you seek hope from something different, a different outcome for the eczematous skin. This is why knowledge is key. There are many people who have moved on from eczema and most are glad to never discuss the topic again. They take whatever knowledge they learned with them. They fail to share the knowledge that allowed them to move on from the manage/maintain mental state.

And that allows me to share the available knowledge. There is the frequently heard medical and social knowledge that holds people in the limited belief that they should prepare for perpetual eczema. Even if the eczema quietens down, they should expect it to return with flares. People who wish to remain constrained by those mental boundaries must be allowed to do so.

They:

- *know* where they are
- *know* what to expect
- *know* how good they are at maintaining eczema
- *know* a lot and may not want to know any more.

I simply offer what one person who moved on from eczema wishes to share. I am content that sufficient people caught in the eczema trap will want to at least look at the knowledge I found very helpful.

There is no right or wrong knowledge. Perhaps we could divide it into helpful and harmful knowledge, yet even that relies on the person's perspective. For a person in the mindset of remaining with eczema, the most helpful knowledge is around which products are best at maintaining the state of inflammation in the skin. To be precise, they learn which products maintain eczema. Obviously they are very unlikely to view it that way. However, if experts they trust tell them to use a certain type of skincare product and the skin remains red and itchy, that knowledge is what they find most helpful.

From a completely different perspective, it becomes valid to ask if that same information is harmful. To see that viewpoint, it is necessary to at least consider that a different outcome is possible: that it is possible for eczematous skin to heal itself. Mine did and the same has happened for many others.

What knowledge did I see Dr Harley and my mother discover when I was a child with constant eczema? What knowledge have I spent my recent years appreciating and reviewing while I was enjoying life with happy, normal skin?

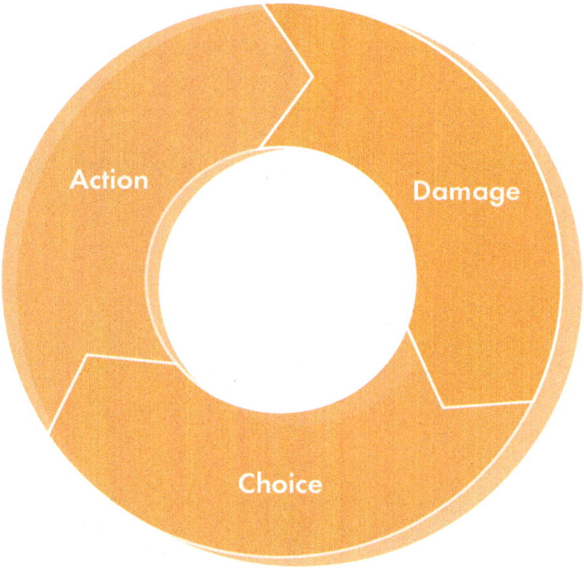

Choice is part of psychology

It is the knowledge that psychology was missing while I suffered from eczema, and it is psychology which has allowed me to remain eczema-free.

It is that clarity of knowledge which you might find is key.

CHAPTER 5

PATHOGENESIS

I will begin this chapter by saying that this may be a challenge for many of my readers to read. I will also remind you that without challenges, no one will ever progress.

I acknowledge it will be tough to read for anyone who switches off at the mention of science. It was even tough for me to understand, and I love science! This chapter details the science behind eczema – why your skin and body react the way they do. It is useful to read it in order to understand the science yourself. But equally, if it proves too difficult, you don't have to force yourself to understand it all. It is merely here to educate those who would like to understand the science themselves.

The skin is an incredibly complicated organ. Yet with explanations and guidance, its complexity can be simplified. Everything it does is rooted in its basic job of keeping our insides in and the outside out. In the process, it constantly utilises physiology.

PHYSIOLOGY

Physiology is the science of life; the branch of biology that aims to understand the mechanisms of living things, from the basis of cell function at the ionic and molecular level, to the integrated behaviour of the whole body and the influence of the external environment.

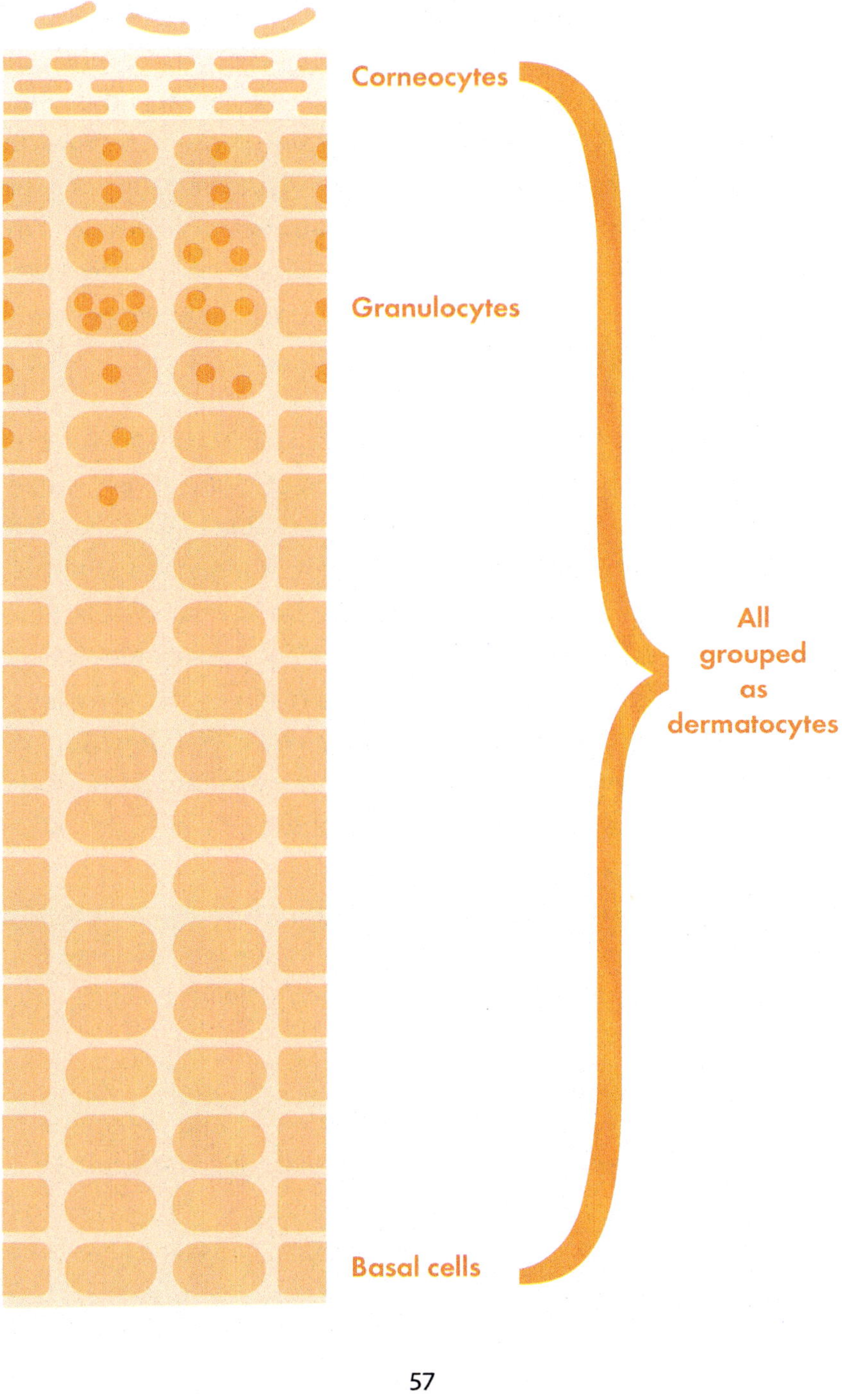
Corneocytes
Granulocytes
All grouped as dermatocytes
Basal cells

If you look down at your hands right now, you will see the very outer layer of skin. This layer is called the epidermis. Very thin, the epidermis layer is usually as thick as a piece of paper. In the elbow and knee folds, this can be even thinner. You may notice how this is where eczema often plagues you the longest. Typically, there are 20 layers of cells making up the epidermis layer in most areas of the body.[15] All 20 layers of these cells are generally given the generic name of dermatocytes. They are then given special names at different stages of their maturation journey.

These names arose long ago when histology was the most advanced way of examining cells. The histologists would look at thin stained layers of tissue under a microscope. They were able to see differences between the cells in various layers, making it logical to apportion special names for what they presumed were specialist cells. Since then, science has been able to determine what is happening at each particular layer. When the original names given by the histologists made sense in relation to the cells' newly discovered function, the name continued to be used. A good example is the granulocytes which the histologists could see contained granules. We know now that the granules contain the material that will be pushed out of the cells to form the extracellular matrix which becomes the moisture-retaining skin barrier layer. So the granulocytes kept their descriptive name since it was a good fit with their function according to physiology.

The bottom-most layer of these 20 layers making up the epidermis is called the basal layer, which contains basal cells. These basal cells divide in the normal cell cycle. The basal cells act as stationary parent cells, with the parent remaining anchored in the basal layer while the newly created progeny cells move upwards through the layers, maturing as they go. These cells are their own factory – each one produces multiple proteins and lipids (fats). In relation to eczema, they produce the filaggrin protein – important for maintaining a strong skin barrier as I mentioned previously – and the ceramide lipid. Eventually, they will fall off the body as dead, dry cells.

In normal, healthy skin, each of the dermatocytes is joined to its neighbours by special bonds called desmosomes.

As they reach the outer layer of the skin, the water is reclaimed from them. This leads to the cells drying, ready to fall off. When they are ready to fall off as dry cells, their usual name is corneocytes. Enzymes break the desmosome junctions so each cell falls apart from one another.[16]

ENZYMOLOGY

Enzymology is the study of enzymes – proteins that catalyse biological chemical reactions – their kinetics, structure, how they fold and function, as well as their relation to each other.

When the dry cells fall off, they are unnoticeable – a single cell is invisible to the human eye as it is so small. However, in damaged, eczematous skin, the enzymes struggle to work properly. The junctions between cells are not broken sufficiently. If any of you are suffering with severe eczema at the moment, look down at it. You may notice there are visible clumps of dry skin that can flake off. This is the consequence of the enzyme not working properly. Dead cells remain attached to each other, which shows as flakes of joined cells.

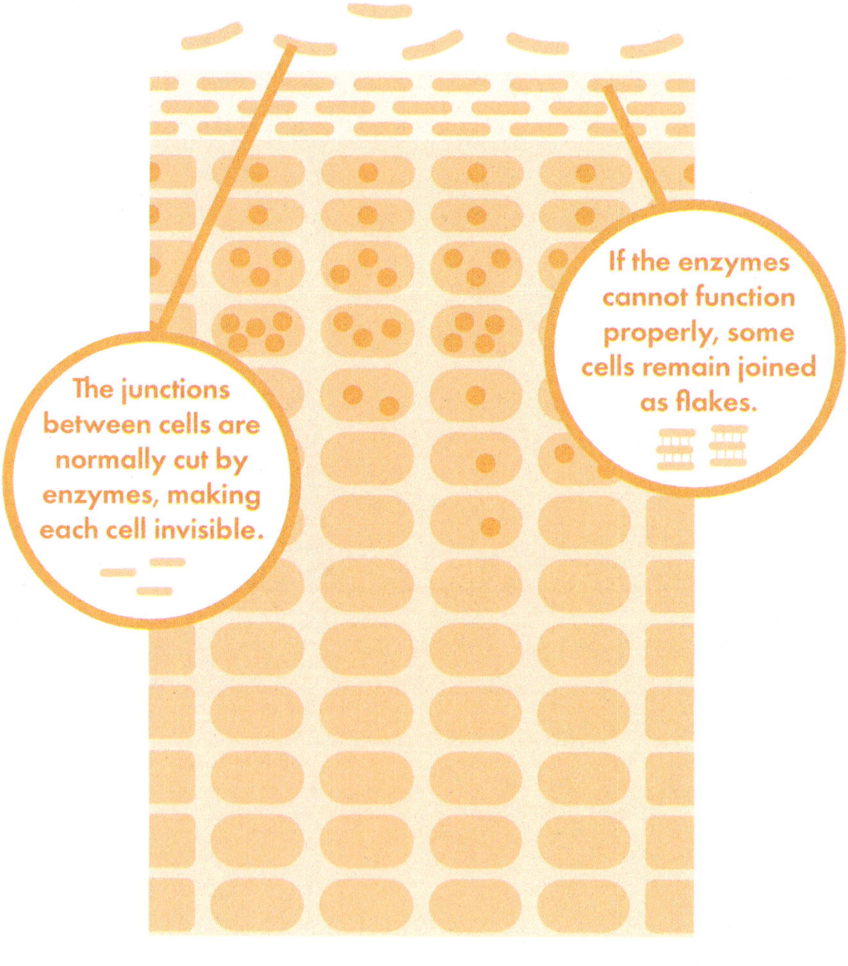

I have also mentioned the skin barrier a lot in previous chapters. Some of you may be wondering, "What actually is the skin barrier? Isn't all the skin a barrier?" Well yes, but scientists can often be very specific in their specialties. The group who discovered the very narrow layer of chemicals which held in the moisture were only thinking of their area of expertise and named the chemical layer the "skin barrier", apparently without considering that all the skin was a barrier. Yet the name they chose has stuck and we are stuck with talking about a skin barrier within a barrier skin. As if it wasn't hard enough already!

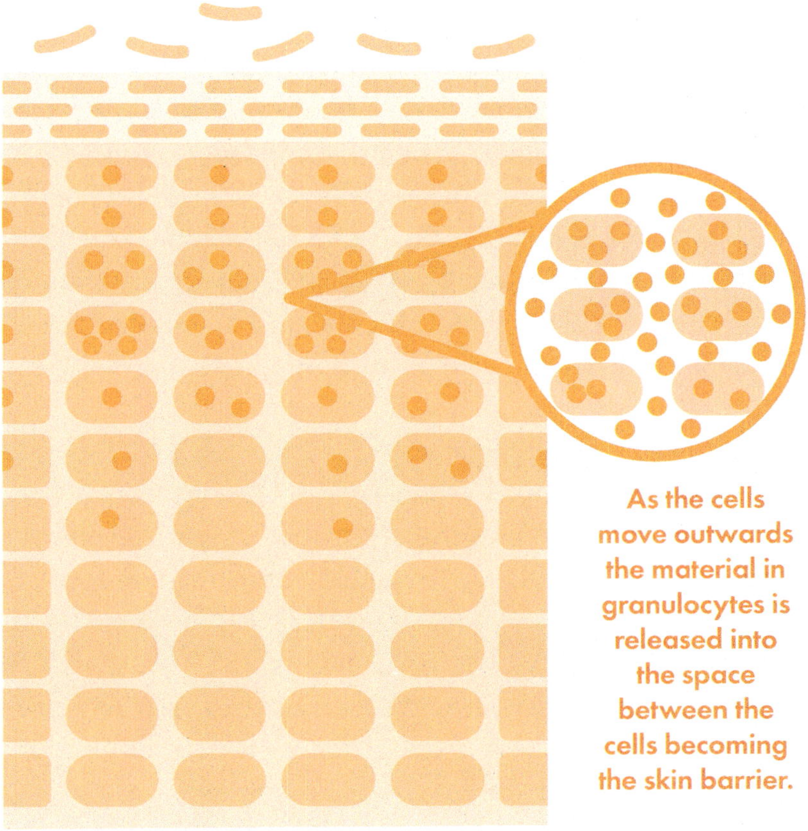

As the cells move outwards the material in granulocytes is released into the space between the cells becoming the skin barrier.

The skin barrier is located in the epidermis just below the surface, a few cell layers deep. It is made up from a combination of the filaggrin protein amino acids and ceramide lipids which have been released from the dermatocytes as they near the outer surface.

The amino acids and ceramide lipid combine in the extracellular space between the cells and together make the skin barrier. The skin barrier will always let some moisture out, and can let more out if it is needed. For example, during times of trouble, the skin barrier will let out more moisture to rid the body from the toxins. This is why the skin barrier needs to be highly sensitive and responsive to the body. During times of stress, we say the skin barrier is less effective in terms of retaining moisture. When you look at this from the *inside view*, you realise it is actually more effective in that one of its jobs is to release moisture. When needed, it lets out more moisture than usual and the affected person senses an area of dry skin. It does this so the "toxins" formed during times of stress can pass out of the body with the moisture. In reality, for the stressed person, it severely dries out their skin. Something I've experienced, this can develop into eczema unless you provide it with appropriate supportive care.

In order to understand eczema best, especially in this chapter called pathogenesis (which means the origin and development of a disease), it's important to realise that the dry skin which usually precedes eczema is a good thing. Dry skin is what Nature intended, and the cells which caused the patch to become dry were performing their natural functions correctly. The dry areas of skin should be there. The dry areas are normal, intended and expected. They may feel horrible and look unfortunate. However, it is what we do to those dry areas that leads to the irritant condition we call eczema.

"... the dry skin which usually precedes eczema is a good thing."

For the skin barrier to function optimally, there needs to be the correct balance of two things: hygroscopic amino acids and ceramide lipids. The amino acids are formed by the filaggrin protein breaking into pieces.[17] They retain water, helping the skin barrier control moisture loss, hence the name hygroscopic. Meanwhile, the ceramide lipids repel water. They are located in such a way that they help the body retain moisture, too. Ceramide lipids form in a double layer – a bilayer. This is relevant to eczema when talking about mineral oils often found in moisturisers, creams and lotions. In the 1992 mineral oil article[12], they found that mineral oils actually penetrate the skin to then reside in between these two layers of ceramide lipids, which can affect their water repelling capability.

When either one of the ceramide lipids or the hygroscopic amino acids are out of this balance – when there is too little of one – the barrier will not be able to retain as much water, leading to moisture loss. Now, releasing more moisture is the correct thing for the body to do when something in the body is abnormal. Eczema is abnormal. The skin barrier releases water. Again, something you may have experienced with your eczema is it becoming oozy, almost wet to touch, when it becomes particularly inflamed (in my experience). This is the skin barrier releasing more water, which the body wants it to do, to flush out abnormalities. The body doesn't want us to have eczema – it is simply protecting us.

"The body doesn't want us to have eczema – it is simply protecting us."

An example of when the amino acids and the ceramide lipids are out of balance is during times of stress. Adrenal glands make cortisol hormone every day. When stressed, the body produces more cortisol than usual. In turn, this reduces the amount of ceramide lipid made by the granulocyte skin cells and so "weakens" the skin barrier. More water can pass out. The person feels this as dry skin. It is really important to repeat that this is normal and the correct response by the skin.

The pharmaceutical industry has been able to manufacture cortisol out of the body, which is what can be in steroid creams. As you undoubtedly know, steroids are found in many products prescribed for eczema use. If you have had reason to manage moderate to severe eczema, you may have used such a product. In fact there are several different types of steroids which is why you hear about "mild" steroids and "stronger" steroids. For our use here I will simply group them as steroids.

Some eczema patients dislike forms of steroid creams containing cortisol, yet this hormone is essential to life. From an eczema sufferer's perspective, putting on cream containing cortisol may be worse than eczema itself. But the response to cortisol is Nature's way of flushing out "toxins" – abnormalities of stress – to protect you. As much as I'm sure you (and I too!) want to blame our bodies for this, Nature has our best in mind. It dries the skin in defence, so it is a valid response. The only thing that needs to change in order to help is the stress. Unfortunately, this, I know, is easier said than done. Eczema relates to something that humans do rather than what Nature designed.

> **"Eczema relates to something that humans do rather than what Nature designed."**

Now we're going to zoom in a little. Inside every cell in the body are genes. Genes are lengths of genetic material which code for specific proteins. Proteins are made in the process of translation, where the gene is read by sub-cellular structures called ribosomes. The ribosomes join amino acids one after the other until the chain of amino acids becomes the specific protein coded for by the gene. Different amino acids chain together in different sequences to form different proteins.

Specifically, dermatocytes follow this process to form a large protein called profilaggrin. When a part of profilaggrin breaks off, the active filaggrin protein is formed. This functional protein helps align keratin molecules (keratin being the protein that forms the main structural constituent of hair, nails and, most importantly, skin). Filaggrin then breaks apart into specific amino acids used to create a functional skin barrier. In essence, the production of profilaggrin is essential.

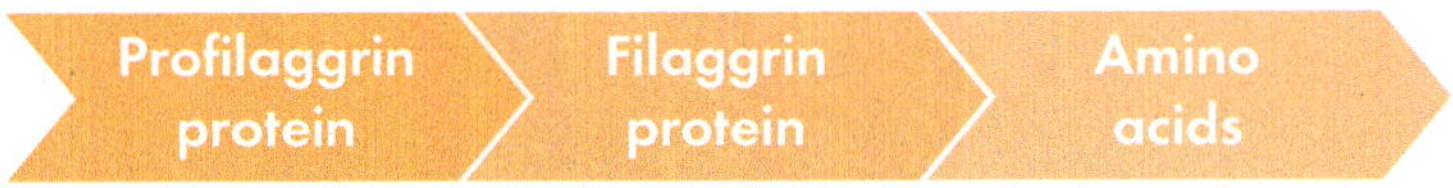

This is why it is so much of a problem when the skin gets inflamed. Inflammation makes it difficult to read the filaggrin gene – no filaggrin protein can be produced.[18]

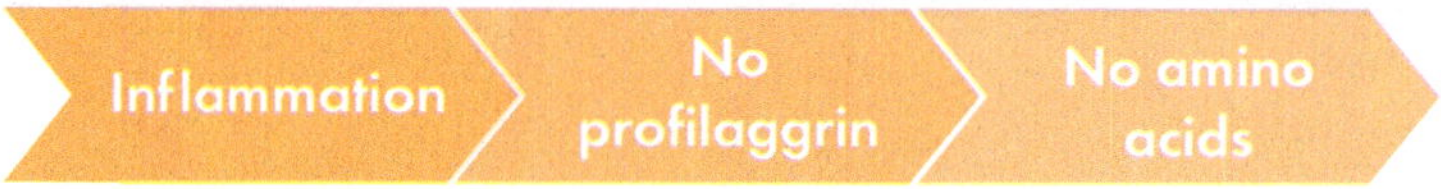

The inflammation can be due to food reactions, infection, contact with an irritant or allergens – the cause is irrelevant. It all has the same effect: minimal filaggrin production. Without filaggrin, there is a suboptimal skin barrier, and so "unnecessary" water loss occurs. That is the perspective used in "normal" eczema thinking, the *outside view*. Using the *inside view*, you know now that this is actually *necessary* water loss because Nature wants the extra outflow of moisture to take toxins with it and help the person.

And by now, halfway into this book, you might be able to figure out where "unnecessary" water loss leads to: dry, cracked skin. Dry skin arises from a weakened skin barrier. Invisible cracks in the epidermis occur long before they can be noticed, from either (or both) reduced ceramide lipids or fewer amino acids in the epidermis. The skin is already dry from Nature attempting to flush away abnormalities. When cracks form, they are much more efficient to expel water from, leading to further loss of water.

In lots of cases, moisturisers are the logical next step. Yet as we now know, many prescribed moisturisers and emollients contain mineral oil, like paraffin or petrolatum. Mineral oil acts as a water repellant to help the skin retain moisture. However, unlike a sheet of plastic kitchen film which would form a waterproof barrier on the skin, mineral oils do not stay on the surface. They penetrate several cells deep into your skin and settle in between the bilayer of ceramide lipids. Consequently, the bilayers separate. Little blisters then form – these are the vesicles (small fluid-filled sacs) mentioned in a few definitions of eczema. If mineral oils cause something that eczema is defined as, then we can say that they are a definitive cause of that aspect of eczema.

With the ceramide lipid bilayer separated, the water repellant properties it gives to the skin barrier are weakened, leaving a suboptimal skin barrier. The sufferer will get dry skin. Normally, dryer skin leads to the application of more emollient. And we only know too well that more emollient often means more mineral oil, which means more dry skin. This is the scientific aspect of the eczema cycle, or eczema trap, I often refer to.

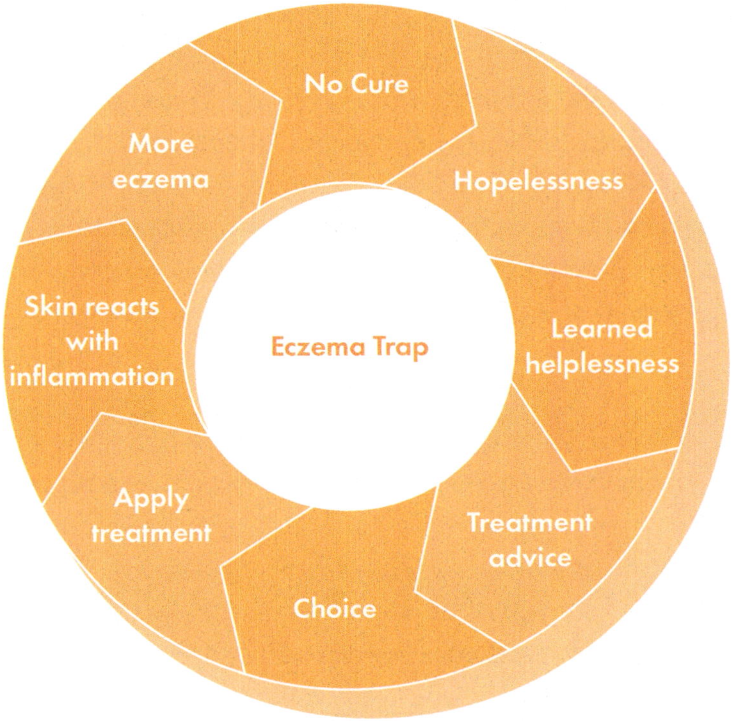
No Cure
Hopelessness
Learned helplessness
Treatment advice
Choice
Apply treatment
Skin reacts with inflammation
More eczema
Eczema Trap

Eczema Trap is a perpetual circle

Mineral oil also passes down cracks in dry skin, resulting in an irritant reaction and inflammation. When the skin is inflamed, it cannot read the gene coding for filaggrin, and so cannot produce filaggrin protein. This leads to water loss and is another cause of another eczema trap.

To reduce this inflammation, often topical steroids are used. This is desirable on a scientific level so that cells are free to produce filaggrin. Some people dislike steroids as they can "thin the skin" due to the cortisol contained in them. A stressed eczematous person will have two sources of cortisol: their own endogenous steroid from their adrenal glands, and the steroid applied as a drug. Both reduce ceramide lipids. And both can arise as a consequence of eczema.

The steroid drugs in topical steroids are most often carried in lipid carriers. Whether the carrier be creams or lotions, they usually contain mineral oil. While the steroid drug is actively reducing inflammation, the mineral oil disrupts the skin barrier. When the steroid wears off, the residual effect of the mineral oil continues. This often leads to the application of more products containing oil. And so this is the pathology of why we remain trapped in an endless cycle of eczema.

I have mentioned that knowledge is key when it comes to eczema. With this knowledge given here, I have provided the opportunity for you to come to a very well-informed choice regarding your skin and how to help your eczema. Some of this was the information given to me and my mother when we first met Dr Harley. And this was the information we collectively used and acted upon in order to heal my skin. It is up to you what you do with this information.

However, it is important to say that some of the facts discussed in this chapter were not known when I was born and also while I suffered from eczema. They were not available, so nobody could have used the knowledge to prevent me developing eczema as a baby. Now we do know the facts, and I share them so everyone can benefit.

Times change and we can change with them.

Staying behind may leave you in eczema misery.

CHAPTER 6

PSYCHOLOGY

There is one key part to having wonderful, eczema-free skin. Listen to it. Countless times before I began my journey to healed skin, I was told "don't scratch". My parents would tell me off for scratching. Obviously they were talking to my mind rather than my skin. Even if I didn't realise it, they were using psychology.

PSYCHOLOGY

Psychology is the scientific study of the mind and how it dictates and influences our behaviour, from communication and memory to thought and emotion.

Now we know the reason that I was scratching was because I was putting creams on my skin, which irritated it. So now, when I feel the urge to scratch, I don't try to ignore it, as that would prove quite impossible in the long run. Instead I listen to it. I find the root of the irritation and try to fix that. This root cause may be a new shower gel, a woolly jumper or even stress, but I will always listen to my skin and remove the irritation. I know I have two choices with diametrically opposed outcomes.

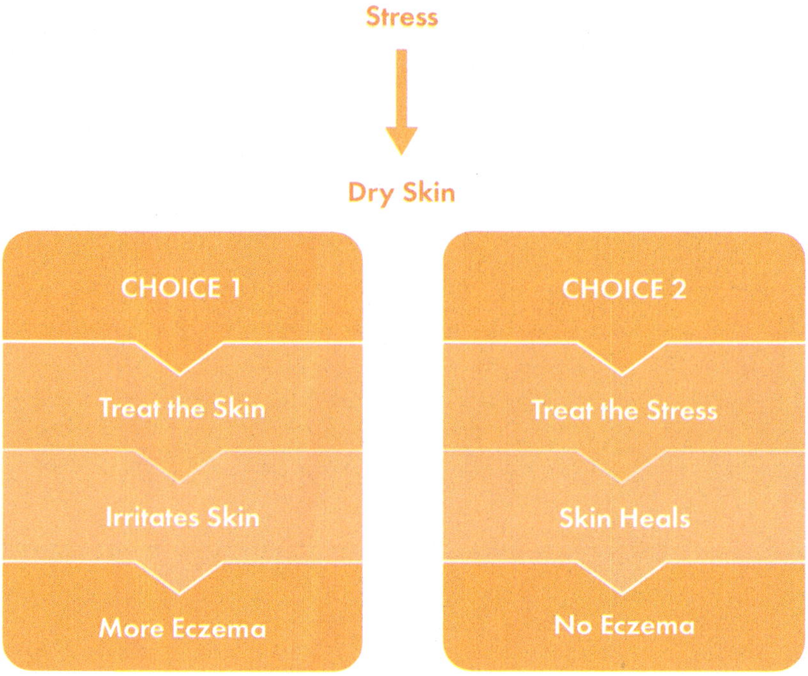
Stress
Dry Skin
CHOICE 1
Treat the Skin
Irritates Skin
More Eczema
CHOICE 2
Treat the Stress
Skin Heals
No Eczema

Choice one, to treat the skin, has long been the only choice. Treating skin and providing advice on treating skin both belong in the domain of medical professionals and particularly dermatologists. Even though I aspire to become a medical doctor, I am currently still at school and clearly not qualified to advise on choice one. Therefore I do not even attempt to do that.

My contribution lies elsewhere. Choice two involves instilling a new mindset which encourages a person to explain eczema. As soon as they can explain eczema, they gain control over it through the choice of doing something different. Choice two involves standard wellbeing coaching methods which are freely available for any person to use. I help people come to their own realisations that another choice is available. If it turns out they are content with what they had before being introduced to this book, then I am happy for them. However, if they have an interest in knowing how the mind affects the skin, then they are likely to gain from the way I explain eczema here.

For the absolute avoidance of doubt, I want to make it perfectly clear that the thrust of this book rests entirely in the mind relating to choice two. Anyone who wishes to utilise the treatment of skin or reinforce that choice is directed to medical professionals who can advise them.

My ideal is to see both choices become equally available. People who wish to treat the skin know who their medical advisers are, what products are being suggested, how to apply them and how often. They are also likely to know what the skin will be like when they do. The choice to follow that path remains open to them, as it should do.

I simply add an additional choice for anyone interested in a new mindset; a choice that involves wellbeing and mental health. Doctors can become involved with the mindset choice, and I eagerly await more doctors directing their thinking and patients to this additional choice in the future.

My ideal is to see both choices become equally available.

Just as doctors used to routinely prescribe antidepressants and now often prescribe wellbeing coaching, I hope *Eczema The inside view* will induce many to move from prescribing emollients and drugs for eczema, and to favour wellbeing coaching.

Genetic factors, like the filaggrin gene defect, often allow for a trap to occur. Being told you have a predisposition to have an ineffective skin barrier, may trap some into resignation that they will forever have eczema. Despite this genetic defect being very valid in terms of increasing the tendency to have eczema, the skin can heal itself of eczema. There have been many known cases in which the irritant is removed and the skin then recovers.

The difference between the two cases is that the people who heal have a different mindset: one of hope, which leads to positive action. They believe their skin can heal. They choose to escape the cycle of maintaining eczema. They give their skin the opportunity to heal itself. Like my own journey to recovery, it was their mindset that changed for the good, allowing them to choose to heal. It was a change in psychology which presented a new choice.

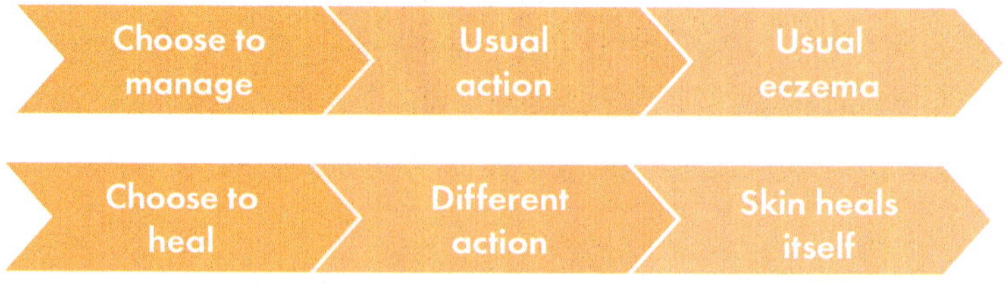

You may also have noticed the improvement in your skin when steroid creams are applied to reduce inflammation. You may also have noticed how I have mentioned them on my lists of prescribed treatments that can make eczema worse. Don't get me wrong, the steroid drugs themselves do an exceptional job of reducing inflammation. But without inflammation, there is no need for steroid creams. And this can simply be achieved by stopping the application of those emollients, lotions and moisturisers that irritate the skin.

As in the name "steroid cream", steroids are mixed with a cream. The steroids themselves work well. But the cream part of steroid creams is still a foreign substance. It can still penetrate the skin barrier and cause irritation. The very creams themselves that are made to carry steroids which reduce inflammation, can also be a contributing factor towards it.

Steroid Cream

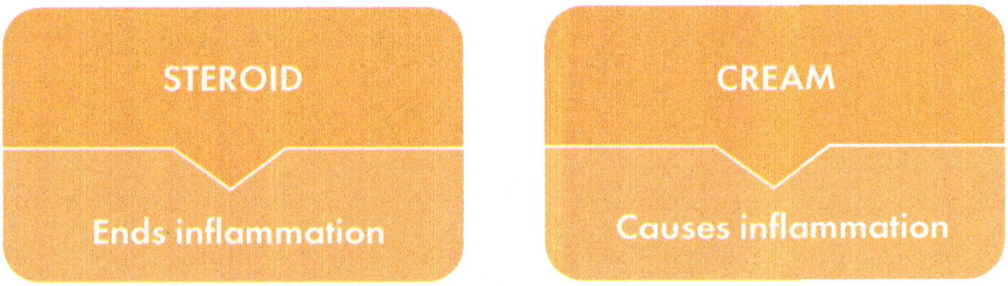

When the steroid wears off the cream
is causing inflammation

By escaping the eczema cycle of maintenance, there will be no need for steroid creams in order to reduce inflammation. There will be no cause of inflammation and therefore no inflammation to reduce.

Numerous people who have the mindset that eczema cannot be cured will be the ones whose eczema will not go away. Atopic eczema can persist in an individual for decades, sometimes forever. While they retain this belief, they will continue to use their prescribed treatments to manage their eczema. They might work on the surface, or in the short run, for example by making their dry skin feel more moisturised. Underneath, however, the new skin cells are being damaged. While they continue to do what they have always done, the eczematous skin will continue to do what it has always done.

The choice on what to apply and when to apply it comes from your mind. Nowhere else. Though doing something different can sometimes be scary, different brings hope. If you are continually applying creams and the skin is continually reacting, nothing will change. It may sound harsh but this is what I have learned myself, the hard way. My mother and I chose to try something different, and it worked. The hope paid off.

Lately I've experienced a first-hand example of how the mind links to eczema. At the beginning of year 11 (GCSE year in England), I noticed dry patches on my elbow. This soon turned into eczema. In hindsight, I know this was due to the subconscious stress of exams. [19] The very real link between the mind and eczema is that when stressed, the body releases the hormone cortisol.

ENDOCRINOLOGY

Endocrinology is the study of hormones. Hormones are essential for our everyday survival. They control our temperature, sleep, mood, stress, growth and more. A hormone is a chemical messenger that travels from one cell to another. Hormones are released in one part of the body, travel in the bloodstream and have an effect on other parts of the body. This helps different parts of the human body to communicate with each other.

The effects of cortisol range widely, but it commonly causes moisture loss in the skin. In essence, it reduces the moisture-retaining ability of the skin barrier. That is the correct and desired protective response intended by Nature. How we choose to react to dry skin is what makes the difference.

"How we choose to react to dry skin is what makes the difference."

I now actively try to reduce stress, as I know it's a cause of my recent eczema (I often found myself scratching without realising; for me it can be the equivalent of biting nails or fiddling with hands – a nervous habit). The point of this story is that the mind is directly connected to your skin. It can be the one thing to heal your eczema. Equally it can be the one thing to cause your eczema. Stress is in the mind, and when allowed to dominate, it leads to dry skin and inflamed skin: eczema.

You could compare it to someone who has smoked their whole life and has recently fallen ill with lung cancer. The addiction is in their mind. Yet the cancer is in their lungs. Cancer is the physical symptom of the addiction.

You could argue that eczema is the physical symptom of a reliance on topical products, like creams. When I was using them, none of us mentioned the word addiction because of its negative connotations. Yet I felt I needed to apply the products multiple times a day, and I knew how horrible my skin would feel if they were not applied at the right time in the right amount. In hindsight it was an addiction, as I feared the effects of not using them.

The mind makes active decisions: to get up, to dress, to shower, to apply shower gel in the shower. The skin reacts accordingly:

- to fight off foreign chemicals in the gel, which have penetrated cracked skin
- to produce an immune reaction against the chemicals that should not be inside the skin

- the immune reaction causes the skin to inflame and itch and to crack even more.

It is a cycle.

There is another way.

The mind makes active decisions: to get up, to dress, to shower, to apply a gentle foam wash. The skin reacts accordingly: if there is no irritant, it continues in its skin cycle. There is no reaction. The skin can heal. The cycle is broken.

The mind and skin are connected. Imagine you arrive at school and someone shouts, "You have your shirt on inside out!" The natural response would be to blush red. The response to the emotion of humiliation (in the mind) results in a change of colour in your face (skin). Not only is the mind connected with eczema, it is connected with all aspects of skin, and your whole body too.

Dr Harley's programme of EXeczema® (EXplain eczema) happens in the mind too. It is made to educate eczema sufferers, and their parents, on the reasons why their skin keeps reacting and the choices they can make. It opens the opportunity for people to choose whether they want to keep doing the same daily routine of applying a concoction of lotions, with the skin doing the same daily routine of reacting and itching; or, it gives them the choice to do different and get different results.

If you are (like I was) applying the same creams every day with the same results and same irritation, the only thing that can break the cycle is different. Different leads to hope. It is your choice to choose different. A simple way to begin is to develop hope. You know now that the best way to satisfy that hope is to begin doing different.

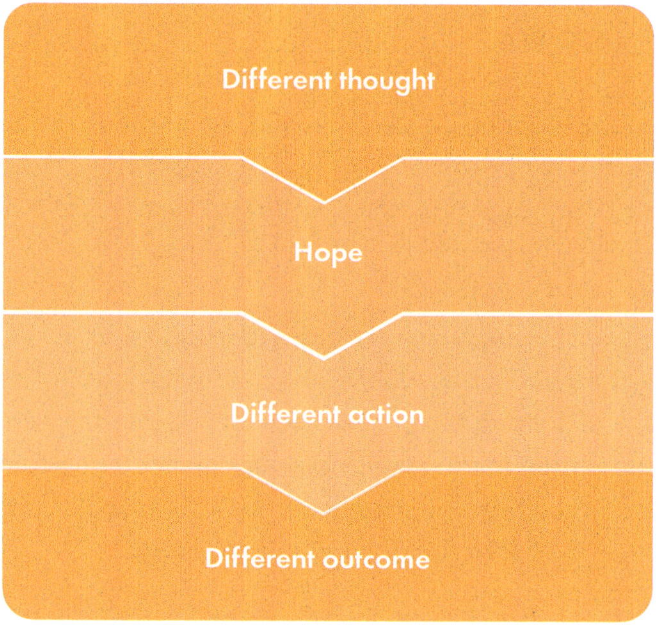

It all begins with a different thought

CHAPTER 7

NUMBERS

From the *outside view*, eczema is all too often about the misery of one single person. Each is an individual with their uniquely personal issues. That's fair and logical, as they each have something terrible to worry about.

From the *inside view*, eczema can be expanded to become a numbers game. There are over six million people in the UK suffering from eczema and that is a large number. There are five times as many in the USA and goodness knows how many in India.

In this book, I aim to point out that every one of those millions share numerous similarities, and by grouping them we can offer help for them all.

140,000 babies alone are diagnosed with eczema within their first year of life – just in the UK. This is a huge figure. I know this great a number may be hard to comprehend, so let me help. Imagine Wembley Stadium, with its tens of thousands of seats. Now imagine a baby with eczema in every one of those seats. To fit every one of the 140,000 babies diagnosed into Wembley, there will have to be 50,000 babies left on the grass. The 90,000 seats are full. Many people who find it challenging to envisage the 140,000 find it easier to comprehend the image of 50,000 babies on the grass. It is horrible and frightening to realise I was one of those babies 17 years ago.

Then appreciate that a new set of 140,000 babies is added every year.

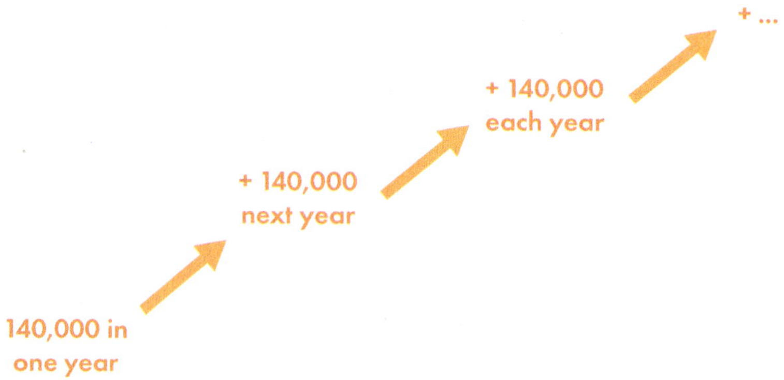

Just picture the magnitude of this problem: every year an additional 140,000 children growing up, their childhood full of doctors and hospital visits, noticeably different to everyone else. And at that point, it is nothing that they have control over. Their lives, their parents' lives, warped out of the norm over something that can be so easily avoided. Unfortunately, I know for so many of you that this will be all too familiar.

The thing is, this figure gets worse. Using age demographics and generally accepted incidence figures, 1.3 million pre-teens and 5 million teens and adults in the UK have eczema. The US has five times the population of the UK, so it's reasonable to say 25 million people in America are suffering. The numbers are imprecise as they're calculated using the fact that 20% of babies have eczema, a number that falls to 10% in the general population. I have seen it stated that there are 36.1 million Americans with eczema. However, do we really care whether it is 25 million or 36.1 million? It is many millions and that is sufficient cause for great concern. And countries where there is increasing disposable income are catching these figures.

Even leaving aside the physical consequences of eczema – the bleeding, the persistent itch, the dry skin, the weeping open wounds which can so easily become infected – there are so many other consequences of eczema.

Mentally, it's been proven that people with eczema are more likely to have a lower quality of life. They can also be more susceptible to psychological diseases like depression or ADHD.[20] This can even affect someone's life so far that the risk of suicidal ideation increases.[21] On top of these devastating potential issues, there are also the financial consequences – from the costs of buying extra or specific items, like clothes and treatments to help with eczema, to even not being able to work and study as efficiently due to the burden of it all. The increasing amount of the world population being diagnosed with eczema will certainly cause an increase in suffering, physically, mentally, financially, and in so many other ways. Something has to be done about it.

As a child with eczema, or a parent of a child with eczema, you might have been dismissed with a "don't worry, they'll grow out of it". My parents were told exactly that. As a child, different to everyone else, it was all I could hope for, that it would magically disappear by itself. Of course, it didn't – not by itself. If you consider the basic maths, you may have put two and two together and realised that most children have not grown out of it: there are still five million teens and adults in the UK with eczema who have most certainly not grown out of it. There's a common belief that 80% of children with eczema do grow out of it. However, if this were true, then only 22% of the 10% of the population with eczema, would have eczema. That's only 2.2%, which conflicts with the generally held figure of 10%.

Similar to conflicting definitions of eczema, conflicting figures lead to confusion. Confusion leads to no action being taken, or even worse, the wrong actions. And in the UK, that leads to over five million people suffering chronically, every day, with eczema.

Personally, I feel that as eczema is not classified as life threatening, some view it as merely a minor skin condition. If you are reading this, then I'm certain you will agree with me when I say that it is anything but that. It is a disease not prioritised to treat. We are dismissed to take care of ourselves, not knowing how to do that. Many people without eczema cannot empathise with eczema sufferers. It has a huge impact on our lives. With colds, the flu, a broken arm, these go away. The person heals. Eczema sufferers wake up every single day with eczema, it does not go away. If anyone is reading this who doesn't have eczema, imagine what that's like. The knock-on consequences of eczema are not well known enough. The view is it's not life threatening, so we can deal with it ourselves.

Think back to 2020/2021 when Covid-19 first hit. Yes, it was a highly contagious disease. But yes, also, the mortality rate was less than 1%. Thousands of hours, millions of people, and billions upon billions of pounds were put into combatting it. Now think of what might happen if just a fraction of that effort could be put into educating both patients and medical professionals about the reality of eczema, and treating it properly, instead of dismissing it as unimportant. So much could be done to help the millions of sufferers.

With the right education and recognition, there wouldn't have to be the 90,000 babies in the seats of Wembley Stadium plus the 50,000 babies left on the grass of Wembley every year. With this book, that is my aim.

CHAPTER 8

MANAGE = MAINTAIN

When it comes to treating eczema, wherever you look, usually the first thing you will see is the word moisturiser. The NHS website, the National Eczema Society website, the NICE treatment flowchart … everything urges us to apply moisturiser. And it makes sense from the *outside view*. With dry skin, the logical thing to do is to apply something that should theoretically stop the dry skin.

Yet it doesn't.

With many cases of atopic eczema, patients apply lotions, emollients and creams every day. Multiple times a day in some cases. I for one can vividly remember during a holiday having to stay at home to be able to keep up with the routine of slathering all types of substances on myself many times a day. In moderate cases, perhaps the bandages and wet wrapping were not as needed, but the lotions and steroid creams would have been. And even in mild cases, most of the time, emollients would still be applied every day.

Each person who has atopic eczema, every one of those millions of sufferers, is different. The only common ground they all share is the fact they have eczema – and use emollients. What if it is certain emollients that are the problem? What if the very things that are supposed to, designed to, and prescribed to heal us, make it worse?

"What if it is certain emollients that are the problem?"

If you're thinking that this is ridiculous, I would urge you to reconsider for one second. If the creams and lotions prescribed did their job, then why are you reading this? Why do you need help with your skin? Shouldn't it have healed? It heals quickly when you graze your knee, so your skin knows how to heal itself. And it does so if nothing stops it from following its natural healing process. So why does it not heal itself with eczema?

"... your skin knows how to heal itself... So why does it not heal itself with eczema?"

The reason is this: dry, eczematous skin has microscopic cracks. The skin is designed to keep the outside out and our insides in. With these cracks, the outside can get in.

Moisturisers are designed in such a way that they form a layer to prevent water escaping, hence keeping your skin moist, and stop it from drying out. But with these microscopic cracks in the skin, that layer of chemicals can get inside your body. The skin has failed to do its job and the outside has got in. Now, the body recognises that this isn't part of yourself and produces an immune reaction against the foreign material in order to expel any danger. Your skin becomes red and itchy.

The red itchy skin gets scratched. The skin becomes damaged and dryer. More moisturiser is put on. More itchiness occurs. Sadly, this is what many of us have gone through for years.

My primary school years were spent applying creams and not questioning why they weren't working, why my eczema would continue getting worse. Where my parents and I thought we were managing my eczema, in reality, we were maintaining it. And this was so proved when Dr Harley introduced us to the science behind eczema and we then stopped applying these creams. Dr Harley and my mother were only working out the specifics at the time, so it took a while for my skin to adjust from the years of harsh chemicals. But in the end, it healed itself. Within a year I was unrecognisable. I know now that my skin suddenly healed within weeks when Dr Harley and my mother finally discovered the secret.

The moisturisers, which should help our skin, actually maintain the misery. That is worth emphasising.

"The moisturisers, which should help our skin, actually maintain the misery."

The pharmaceutical industry cannot be blamed, though. These creams would work perfectly well on healthy skin. Skin that has an optimally functioning skin barrier would be less able to absorb the chemicals. The waterproof layer would stay fully active upon the surface of the skin and help the skin keep its moisture in order to prevent dryness. It would moisturise. It is just the unlucky fact that the people who truly need these products are the ones who cannot use them. The fact that mineral oils are damaging has been known for years, however. The evidence was published in 1992 before I was born. Yet they are still being prescribed, apparently without a second thought.

"It is just the unlucky fact that the people who truly need these products are the ones who cannot use them."

It is because some creams *tell* the skin what to do. Topical steroids tell the body to suppress the immune reaction. Mineral oils tell the skin that it must keep its moisture – it has no other choice, as the layer it creates is hydrophobic (water repellant). So the products suppress the very immune reaction and moisture loss that Nature uses to heal us. The products keep eczema sufferers in a state of unnatural imbalance. It's what Dr Harley calls Product Maintained Dermatitis in his iatrogenic article.[1]

What we need, what the skin needs, are products that *allow* the skin to heal and return to its natural, balanced state. From there our skin can do what it was made for, the thing it has evolved over hundreds of thousands of years to do: protect us.

The outer epidermis layer of the skin fully replaces itself every month. In natural conditions, it will have had a chance to completely heal and repair itself in that month, on its own. If you are using a treatment and the eczema is still there after that month, it is wise to assume that it is the treatment that is the problem. That is, if no other factors are affecting your skin, like stress, diet or clothing. By keeping these other factors at an optimum, you will be able to determine whether the treatment is working, or whether it is maintaining your eczema.

Unfortunately, you'll soon come to realise, most of the time the answer is that it is part of the problem.

We all know that eczema, physically, is horrible. The itch, the angry, flaming skin and the weeping, open wounds. That in itself is horrible enough to deal with. What I would like to open up is the knock-on effects of eczema, the less talked about side of the disease. To put this into perspective, I'll list some statistics:

•Children and adolescents with atopic eczema are two to six times more likely to have depression, anxiety or conduct disorder than children without eczema.[22]

•Sleep disturbance occurs in approximately 60% of children with eczema, and parents of children with eczema are four to eight times more likely to average less than six hours of sleep per night compared with caregivers of healthy children.[23]

•Recent studies have suggested people with eczema are up to 44% more likely to exhibit suicidal ideation, and 36% are more likely to attempt suicide.[24]

•One-third to one-half of adults with eczema avoid social interactions because of their appearance.[25]

Not many people, unless you've suffered with it first hand, know that eczema, mentally, is horrible, too.

The world is beginning to open its eyes and become much more accepting around ill mental health. So much more is being done to help everyone. There are:

- assemblies in schools
- free chatlines
- encouragements to rest.

Society is much more open and understanding nowadays. That's not to say, though, that it has eased the problem. Like eczema, mental health problems are becoming much more rife in the population, and similarly again, rising in young people. I'm sure that many of you will have experienced some ill mental health of varying degrees at some point in your lives, whether it be linked to eczema or not. I'm not saying the rise in mental health problems is due to the rise in eczema. Yet, I believe there is a correlation. As part of managing the mental health problems of the eczema sufferers, why not combat the likely root of the problem: the eczema? That's something we know how to do.

The prevalence of childhood eczema has steadily increased from 8% to ~12% since 1997.[26]

Eczema prevalence has increased and is still increasing. If it hasn't affected you in a negative way, it could affect your friend, neighbour, or your own child in the future. The way to prevent this is to act now.

There are staggering financial and economic effects of eczema too:

- Nearly 5.9 million workdays annually in the US are lost due to eczema.[27]
- The annual economic burden of eczema, including direct medical costs, indirect costs from lost productivity, and quality of life impacts, is conservatively estimated at $5.3 billion.[28]

It is not just those of us with eczema who are suffering; it is the world and its economy. Eczema affects us on a personal level: the itch, the embarrassment, the misery. But it also affects the world as a whole. Think about the extreme amount of money we could save if suddenly eczema wasn't a thing any more. Estimates of the cost to end world hunger range from $7 billion to $265 billion per year. By magically ending eczema, we could make an excellent start on that.

There is also a strong environmental effect. Every product applied to the outside of every eczema sufferer is washed off at some stage, so it goes down the drain into the water system. Every container emptied in the process of managing eczema needs to be considered in the global environmental impact of packaging. By ending eczema, this would be improved too.

Obviously there will be no magic cure to eczema while the *outside view* of eczema prevails. It is mental strength, education and Nature that help the skin begin to heal. Even if I help just one person to help their skin, and so help their mind, their sleep, their lifestyle, their productivity, I will be happy. But with helping one comes another, and another, and another. And in the next chapter, I will demonstrate how we can help them all.

We have the answers that the doctors are either ignoring or are simply unaware of. It has to be down to us.

"It has to be down to us."

CHAPTER 9

COMMUNITY SUPPORT

One of the best memories I have of my eczema support group is when I was riding around the county for a charity bike ride. At just age eight, I felt enormous amounts of pride talking about this event, getting sponsored, the strong sense of family while I made my way round the course with likeminded people. It was the first time I felt I could talk about eczema to others without getting pitied. By then my eczema was gone and my skin was in balance with Nature and me. I felt powerful.

Normally, I would be embarrassed to talk about my eczema. At school, I was the odd one out. I couldn't go round to friends' houses due to my life-consuming routine of creams. I couldn't wear what everyone else was wearing, to minimise irritation. I couldn't wear my hair up – my mother said it looked too greasy, a result of slathering on moisturisers. This is the smallest thing, but to me, the thing that stuck with me the most. Every aspect of your life changes with eczema. And I'm sure, as you're reading this book, you can fully empathise.

I'm going to bring it back to Wembley. The number of babies diagnosed with eczema during their first year of life fills up every seat of Wembley Stadium. And there are still 50,000 babies left on the grass. Yes, a small proportion of these babies do grow out of eczema. By the time they begin nursery or primary school, they are healthy enough for it to go unnoticed. Except, for the vast majority of the 140,000 children, the harsh truth is that they don't grow out of it. Most are like me, and perhaps even you, who grew up suffering with a miserable skin condition; not threatening enough to get urgent support, but severe enough to affect every aspect of our lives and upbringing.

"And there are still 50,000 babies left on the grass."

According to generally accepted statistics, on average there will be 10% of children in a classroom with eczema. In a class of 50 children, that will mean five have eczema. Five more people sharing the same feelings of misery and embarrassment as you and I once felt, and possibly you are still experiencing. So why did I feel so isolated and alone when I was suffering?

The answer is education, or rather the lack of.

I did not know anywhere near as much as I could have done about the complex skin condition that I was suffering from. To be truthful with you, it is only while writing this book that I am discovering some of the really useful information for the first time. Until now, I did not know that eczema, asthma and hay fever went hand in hand. I did not know how the hormones associated with stress can dry the skin.

I did not even know that eczematous skin has microscopic cracks in it. Back then, all I knew was that eczema was itchy and I had to try to stop scratching it for it to go away. Of course, it didn't.

Without this information I couldn't explain what was wrong with me to anyone. If people asked, all I could say was that it was called eczema. People thought I was a freak. They couldn't help me, or even sympathise with me. I was alone. *We* were alone.

"They couldn't help me, or even sympathise with me."

As I've mentioned, the purpose of writing this book is, yes, to help people. But equally to educate people. It is proven that children, adolescents and young adults with eczema often feel isolated from their peers due to disease-related lifestyle restrictions. If the whole concept of eczema was talked about and normalised to the same extent as it is prevalent amongst the population, I would never have been so lonely. My peers would have understood. My teachers would have been able to help me.

The main thing, though, is that I had no idea how common it was. I did go to a very small primary school, but even so, according to the figures, many more people would have had the same condition. And I had no idea. *They* had no idea about me. We were all so squashed down and hidden, we never had the chance to come together.

"We were all so squashed down and hidden …"

I hope to emphasise how common this disease truly is. Yes, it's devastating and something needs to be done to combat it, instead of ignoring and managing it. But, there will be so many more people than you think with atopic eczema, feeling the same way as you do, and as I did: isolated, humiliated, frustrated. With the knowledge that it's so common, we can come together and talk about our experiences, share what worked for us, and empathise with each other.

It is time to act, as it's up to all of us to do what we can to end eczema. This book is intended to make it more likely. Sometimes it helps to show people how becoming involved as individuals can build into global momentum.

"It is time to act, as it's up to all of us to do what we can to end eczema."

When you seek the assistance and collaboration of people who may not know you personally, it is both polite and wise to ensure they can join easily and without untoward challenges. Since this book is all about how to end eczema quickly and permanently, it is vital to ensure everyone knows that this is not a medical claim. Certain authorities have a duty to prevent people making medical claims, and we like to follow their guidelines and advice.

In that regard, it helps to reframe atopic eczema as a mental health condition. It then falls into the category of other common conditions with a mental health component, for example:

- Just as we do now in helping people with obesity and the fear or reality of type 2 diabetes; we correct their mind's appreciation of inappropriate food intake rather than attempt to correct the pancreas. The pancreas will usually return to normal when the root cause in the mind is addressed.
- Just as when we are helping a smoker avoid the dangers of lung cancer; we address their mental addiction to cigarettes rather than treat the lungs. Pre-cancerous cells are usually removed in the lungs when the initiating chemical insults are no longer being inhaled.
- Similarly when we are attempting to help a person move on from eczema; we address their reliance on certain irritant skincare products rather than treat the skin. The skin will return to normal by itself when the irritating chemicals are removed.

" ... it helps to reframe atopic eczema as a mental health condition."

As a school student, I would normally hesitate to suggest how a head teacher should manage mental health in their school. Yet I know how hard they work to reduce the many contributing factors that combine into their challenge. Of all those factors, eczema is likely to be the only one they can eliminate throughout their school within a month. Yes it takes courage and good cross-discipline communication. Yet by using the *inside view*, they can cause it to happen.

During my time with eczema, I met many doctors who, I believed, did not like me having eczema. Yet they were constrained by being told to always use the *outside view* of eczema, so they advised that I apply all those products to my outside. When those doctors come to utilise the *inside view* presented here, they will have a new tool. Their old one didn't end eczema because it so often maintained eczema. The new tool of thinking with the *inside view* does allow them to end eczema. That would greatly improve the average day for so many doctors around the world.

My mother speaks of the many discussions she had with other parents whose children had eczema. Because it was the only option available at the time, they shared ideas from the *outside view*:

- What products were being applied to the outside?
- Which magic pyjamas were best?
- How do you stop your child scratching the itchy patches?
- How do you feel when you see blood on your child's sheets in the morning?

Now my mother can have completely different discussions using the *inside view*. It is acceptable to talk about enhancing mental health and wellbeing. That is less likely to build resentment compared to asking about an abhorrent skin condition that just won't go away.

When the discussion arises from the *inside view*, everything changes and becomes far easier.

In an ideal world, everyone would hear about this book or, at least, its contents:

- why eczema lasts so long
- how common it is
- what eczema actually is.

Children with eczema, instead of being the odd ones out, can band together and help one another through it. Instead of lasting for years, for lifetimes sometimes, eczema will only last until the skin has gone through its skin cycle and healed itself, as people would know how to protect their skin. That cycle only takes a month. Imagine a world where eczema has become so talked about that an eight-year-old child could educate their peers on how to heal their new, itchy rash. I wish I'd had the opportunity to do that. I bet you wish that someone had had the opportunity to say that to you.

So why don't you do it for someone else? I've written this book in the hope that this new world can become a real place. I've provided the education and knowledge needed to do so. It is with this that something different to our long routines of creams begins, and hope is found and spread.

Imagine the feeling of simply repeating words to your friend and changing their life. Nelson Mandela once said that, "Education is the most powerful weapon which you can use to change the world." I wholeheartedly agree. The mere thought of the world being an eczema-free place is so utopian to me. Yet, it is fully plausible. Dr Harley and my mother began the process with one person: me. Since then, there have been many more who have learned to appreciate the *inside view* and end eczema. Through the power of communication, we can help the children and adults alike who have spent too long suffering with cracked, weeping elbows, relentless itching, their eczema getting in the way of their life.

You are one person. Which other one person can you help by introducing them to the *inside view*, either verbally or by providing them with a copy of this book? There are millions who can benefit, and starting with one means you have started.

We only have one life to live. I would hate to see it consumed with eczema. I hate to see anyone consumed with eczema. Now let's help to make this vision of an eczema-free world become reality.

BIBLIOGRAPHY

1. Farmer H. "Is atopic eczema iatrogenic?" *J Alt Comp Med.* (2013); 19:681–3.

2. Farmer H. *What is eczema? A path to ending the misery*. 2nd edition (2016). Published by NewGenn Ltd, UK, NR16 2SR.

3. British Association of Dermatologists https://www.skinhealthinfo.org.uk/condition/atopic-eczema/ (2021).

4. National Eczema Society https://eczema.org/information-and-advice/types-of-eczema/atopic-eczema/ (2021).

5. British Association of Dermatologists Patient Information Leaflets "ATOPIC ECZEMA" https://www.bad.org.uk/patient-information-leaflets/atopic-eczema/?showmore=1&returnlink=https%3a%2f%2fwww.bad.org.uk%2fpatient-information-leaflets#.YYUfrL3Poqo (2021).

6. Cambridge Dictionary entry for eczema https://dictionary.cambridge.org/dictionary/english/eczema (2021).

7. Wadonda-Kabondo N, Sterne JA, Golding J, Kennedy CT, Archer CB, Dunnill MG; ALSPAC Study Team. "Association of parental eczema, hayfever, and asthma with atopic dermatitis in infancy: birth cohort study." *Arch Dis Child*. (2004 Oct); 89(10):917–21.

8. Palmer CN, Irvine AD, Terron-Kwiatkowski A, Zhao Y, Liao H, Lee SP, et al. "Common loss-of-function variants of the epidermal barrier protein filaggrin are a major predisposing factor for atopic dermatitis." *Nat Genet.* (2006 Apr); 38(4):441–6.

9. Smith FJ, Irvine AD, Terron-Kwiatkowski A, Sandilands A, Campbell LE, Zhao Y, et al. "Loss-of-function mutations in the gene encoding filaggrin cause ichthyosis vulgaris." *Nat Genet.* (2006 Mar); 38(3):337–42.

10. Glatz M, Polley E, Simpson E, Kong H. "Emollient therapy alters skin barrier and microbes in infants at risk for developing atopic dermatitis." *J Invest Dermatol.* (2015); 135:S31.

11. The BMJ https://www.bmj.com/content/339/bmj.b2433 (2021).

12. Ghadially R, Lalkier-Sorensen L, Elias PM. "Effects of petrolatum on stratum corneum structure and function." *J Am Acad Dermatol.* (1992); 26: 387–396.

13. National Eczema Society https://eczema.org/information-and-advice/types-of-eczema/atopic-eczema/ (2021).

14. UK Parliament. CHAPTER 2: "The Nature of Allergy" https://publications.parliament.uk/pa/ld200607/ldselect/ldsctech/166/16605.htm (2021).

15. Yousef H, Alhajj M, Sharma S. "Anatomy, Skin (Integument), Epidermis" https://www.ncbi.nlm.nih.gov/books/NBK470464/ (2021).

16. International Association for Applied Corneotherapy https://www.corneotherapy.org/articles/259-enzymes-in-the-body (2021).

17. Brown SJ, McLean WH. "One remarkable molecule: filaggrin." *J Invest Dermatol.* (2012); Mar;132(3 Pt 2):751-62. doi: 10.1038/jid.2011.393. Epub 2011 Dec 8. PMID: 22158554; PMCID: PMC3378480.

18. Howell MD, Kim BE, Gao P, Grant AV, Boguniewicz M, Debenedetto A, et al. "Cytokine modulation of atopic dermatitis filaggrin skin expression." *J Allergy Clin Immunol.* (2007); 120:150–155.

19. Medical News Today https://www.medicalnewstoday.com/articles/eczema-and-stress#summary (2021).

20. Yaghmaie P, Koudelka CW, Simpson EL. "Mental health comorbidity in patients with atopic dermatitis." *J Allergy Clin Immunol.* (2013); 131(2):428–433.

21. Patel KR, Immaneni S, Singam V, Rastogi S, Silverberg JI. "Association between atopic dermatitis, depression, and suicidal ideation: A systematic review and meta-analysis." *J Am Acad Dermatol.* (2019); 80(2):402–410.

22. Yaghmaie P, Koudelka CW, Simpson EL. "Mental health comorbidity in patients with atopic dermatitis." *J Allergy Clin Immunol.* (2013); 131(2):428–433.

23. Chamlin SL, Mattson CL, Frieden IJ, et al. "The price of pruritus: sleep disturbance and cosleeping in atopic dermatitis." *Arch Pediatr Adolesc Med.* (2005); 159(8):745–750.

24. Sandhu JK, Wu KK, Bui TL, Armstrong AW. "Association Between Atopic Dermatitis and Suicidality: A Systematic Review and Meta-analysis." *JAMA Dermatol.* (2019); 155(2):178–187.

25. Silverberg JI, Gelfand JM, Margolis DJ, et al. "Patient burden and quality of life in atopic dermatitis in US adults: A population-based cross-sectional study." *Ann Allergy Asthma Immunol.* (2018); 121(3):340–347.

26. Silverberg JI. "Public Health Burden and Epidemiology of Atopic Dermatitis." *Dermatol Clin.* (2017); 35(3):283–289.

27. Silverberg JI. "Health Care Utilization, Patient Costs, and Access to Care in US Adults With Eczema: A Population-Based Study." *JAMA Dermatol.* (2015); 151(7):743–752.

28. Drucker AM, Wang AR, Li WQ, Sevetson E, Block JK, Qureshi AA. "The Burden of Atopic Dermatitis: Summary of a Report for the National Eczema Association." *J Invest Dermatol.* (2017); 137(1):26–30.

EPILOGUE

I hope this book has provided you with the incentive to invest in a new mindset regarding eczema. If so, you will be ready to end eczema within weeks and without drugs. You will have noticed an absence in the text of any suggestions on how you actually end the eczema. That's because, increasingly, any printed book starts to become redundant the day it is published. Since I believe *Eczema. The inside view* will trigger rapid changes in how people relate to atopic eczema, it is essential that this book keeps pace with the latest changes.

Therefore I have provided the QR code below. When you scan that code, you will be directed to what I consider to be the most useful content available at the time. The code will remain the same, whereas the place it takes you to will change.

Please feel free to contact me via bethanamblin.com with any comments and suggestions you would like to share.

ABOUT THE AUTHOR

Bethan Amblin first struggled with eczema at 18 months old. She grew up trying every technique she had heard of to manage it, with no success - until she was introduced to a new way of thinking. With a change of mindset, her life consumed with eczema soon changed too.

She has the knowledge and experience to manage her own skin now and wants to use this to change others' lives. Out of everyone, she knows just how it feels to be trapped in the eczema cycle.

Inspired by her trips to dermatologists in hospitals, Bethan wants to become a Doctor herself. She wants to use her experiences as a tool to help her empathise with her patients.

In her (precious few moments of) spare time Bethan enjoys athletics and baking.

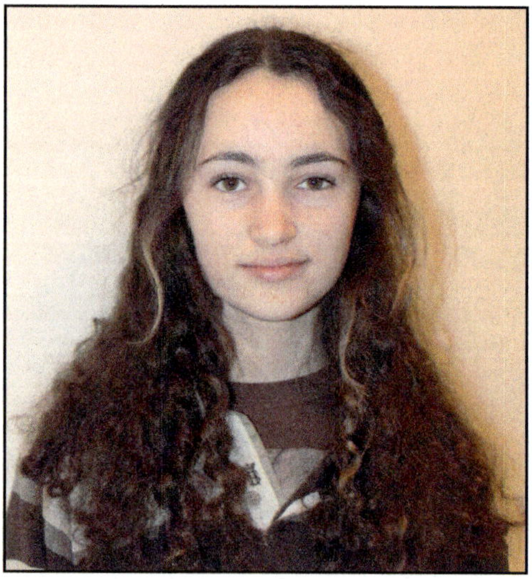

Printed in Great Britain
by Amazon

81941915R00068